# WHAT IS MY CHILD `

# THAT I'M NOT GETTING ...*YET?*

*How to help your baby meet their milestones*

*Learn about your child's Baby Body Language*

*A Guide to Problem-Solving Your Child's Challenges*

## Anne Matthews

BSc Hons (Physiotherapy), DC (Chiropractic), Dip Biomech, FBCA, FCC, CST, PPN Ed

Author & Speaker; Pre & Perinatal Educator; Baby Body Language Expert; Chiropractor; Physiotherapist & Craniosacral Therapist

Foreword by Karlton Terry, world-renowned Baby Therapist

First Published in 2023 by Anne Matthews
with Russell-Alexander Publishing

www.russellalexanderpublishing.com

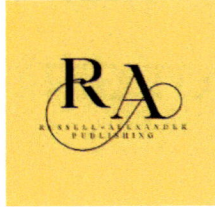

ISBN: 978-1-7395350-0-1

# Dedication

**To the parents who seek a wholesome connection with their children.**

# Contents

Testimonials                                          vi

About the Author                                      vii

From The Prophet                                      xii

Foreword                                              xiii

Introduction                                          xv

Prologue                                              23

Hello and Welcome to my Treatment Room                27

Chapter One                                           31

   Creating a Safe Space               31

Chapter Two                                           63

   Pacing a Child and their Parents    63

Chapter Three                                         105

   Building Trust and Rapport          105

Chapter Four                                          121

   From the Baby's Perspective         121

Chapter Five                                          145

   Supporting the Newborn              145

Chapter Six                                           165

   Integrating Therapies for Children  165

Chapter Seven                                         205

   Challenging Behaviours              205

Chapter Eight                                         219

   Supporting and Guiding Parents      219

Chapter Nine                                          237

   Soulful Connection                  237

Epilogue                                              259

Return                                                283

# Testimonials

*"I cannot recommend Anne and her team highly enough. Our children love her and we love her and we are so grateful to her for all of her care and support to us as a family."*

**Mary Mullin, patient's parent**

*"Anne Matthews is a masterful facilitator. In creating a safe space and modelling the very techniques she intends to impart; she provides a profound education in the effects of pre and perinatal trauma, the power of self-regulation, and the importance of relationship building in facilitating change. The process of Baby Body Language is clear and codified and the course proceeded with presence and flexibility. Anne gives you permission to trust your intuition and invites you to expand your observations and tools. Her online course was enlightening and accessible, as helpful for me and my child as it will be for my patients."*

**Dr. Faraneh Carnegie-Hargreaves, DC. USA**

*"Beginning and ending life...a continuum that entails events that imprint us and influence the next steps on our journey. Anne Matthews' Baby Body Language initiates the "conversation" that often needs to take place between a patient's mind, heart and body and the experiences that are "remembered" by the body (even if the memory has been deeply buried) so that they may heal. The study of epigenetics has shown us the effects that trauma can play in how we manifest our potential. Baby Body Language consists of a set of tools to facilitate the patient's ability to connect their earliest experiences with an understanding of their history and how to release, restore balance physically and emotionally, heal and move on.*

*Anne weaves an understanding of pre and perinatal experiences, neurology and therapeutic technique into her seminar using storytelling, experiential exercises and practical, clinical case presentations to promote a permission-based practice model for practitioners of all health care fields to better serve their patients/clients by being present, being curious and being open to the process that might unfold.*

**Dr Sharon Vallone, DC, KIDSPACE Adaptive Play & Wellness, USA**

# About the Author

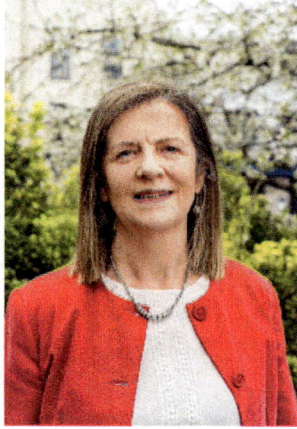

Anne Matthews lives in Belfast and is Clinic Director of the Belfast Chiropractic Clinic and Complementary Therapies which she established formally in 1988. Passionate and enthusiastic about her professional work, Anne is extremely privileged to be part of the lives of thousands of families who have sought her professional help to move through vulnerable and difficult times. It is her absolute pleasure to watch children grow and develop into very capable individuals, sometimes despite early challenges.

Anne is a mum of three, all now adults; she grew with and learned from her children as she established her practice, and expanded her knowledge as a mum, daughter, sister and holistic practitioner focused on pre and perinatal education (PPN Ed), treatment and care.

At the Clinic, Anne has brought together a collaborative care team of natural healthcare practitioners and therapists focusing on the integrative ethos of caring for the diverse needs of the family with the mission of creating wholesomely connected families. She works with newborns and older babies, children, pregnant mums and parents. Her passion is to integrate and weave her therapeutic skills in working with children as a Pre & Perinatal Educator. Anne focuses on the resolution of prenatal, birth and early trauma as she interprets early imprints from the Baby Body Language a baby or child expresses physically, developmentally and emotionally. During a treatment session, Anne facilitates parents to connect in a more heartfelt and soulful way with their child.

Now for the official bit - Anne Matthews, BSc Hons (Physiotherapy), DC (Chiropractic), Dip Biomech, FBCA, FCC, CST, PPN Ed is an independent holistic-based chiropractor with over 36 years of clinical experience. Her professional background includes Physiotherapy, Chiropractic, Biomechanics, Craniosacral Therapy together with Paediatric Neurodevelopmental training. Anne is also a Pre & Perinatal Educator (PPN Ed) having completed the certification programme with the Association for Parental and Perinatal Psychology and Health (APPPAH).

Her interest in PPN Ed work followed on from Craniosacral Therapy and Visceral Manipulation courses taken through the Upledger and Barral Institutes (UK and Ireland) together with the Fascial Release work taught by Carol Phillips, DC (USA). Anne has studied in Europe under the instruction of Karlton Terry, Institute of Pre & Perinatal Education (PPN Ed - USA) for which she has certification in the beginner, intermediate and advanced classes involving hundreds of hours of residential workshops over many years. These included intense birth trauma resolution work involving personal PPN regressions and follow-up mentoring work. She has also completed Ray Castellino's Womb Surround training with Cherionna Menzam-Sills, UK and is a Mentor with APPPAH.

Anne has created and developed her Baby Body Language teaching approach to facilitate an understanding of the PPN Education perspectives in the physical, emotional and developmental challenges of the growing baby and child.

Anne delivers accessible Baby Body Language workshops to parents, practitioners, therapists and teachers in Europe and the USA. A dedicated lifelong learner, she keeps up to date with the latest research in these fields of study.

Having worked in hospital settings in both the UK and Ireland and as an independent practitioner since 1986, her practice protocols reflect the current professional standards of good practice as outlined by the statutory and regulatory bodies to which she belongs. Her professional work is underpinned by current evidence-based research in the areas of child development, chiropractic, craniosacral therapy and pre and perinatal education.

Anne will be offering online health coaching courses for parents as a Baby Body Language expert and Pre and Perinatal Educator at www.WholesomelyConnected.com

## Disclaimer 1: Family Units

I want to acknowledge the many different types of loving family units from the idea of the traditional family of mum, dad and baby to the families of a single parent, same-sex parents, those children who live with adoptive or foster parents and those children who have full, half-siblings or step-siblings. I want to acknowledge the babies who have been conceived naturally, those born from a surrogate mum or gestational carrier and those whose conceptions were assisted. I respect gender identity.

The developing interrelationships between parents, children and the extended family are very complex and need to be considered on a case-by-case basis. For ease of writing and for the purpose of this book in which I will be developing the concepts of Baby Body Language, particularly from the child's perspective, I will be referring to the family as parents or the mum and dad and using the male and female pronouns. Please adjust as befits your family and experience.

## Disclaimer 2: Professional advice

This book provides some tips and tools within the guidance sections at the end of each chapter. These are not a substitute for professional medical advice. If you intend to engage with a professional in this field then, before using any of the tools within this book, please consult your physician or mental health professional, if you have one, and show them the tools that you are looking to use or incorporate.

All the case studies contained within this book are from the testimony of actual clients. All names and some details have been changed to protect client identity. If you find any of the contents within this book or case studies challenging, please do seek professional support.

## Disclaimer 3: Information is general

Neither the publisher nor the author is engaged in rendering professional advice, or services, to the individual reader. The ideas, procedures and suggestions contained in this book are not intended as a substitute for consulting with your doctor. All matters regarding your health require medical supervision.

Neither the author nor the publisher will be liable or responsible for any loss or damage allegedly arising from any information or suggestions in this book.

# From The Prophet

### Kahlil Gibran

*"Your children are not your      children*

*They are the sons and daughters of life's longing for itself*

*They come through you but not from you*

*And though they are with you, yet they belong not to you*

*You may give them your love but not your thoughts*

*For they have their own thoughts*

*You may house their bodies but not their souls*

*For their souls' dwell in the house of tomorrow..."*

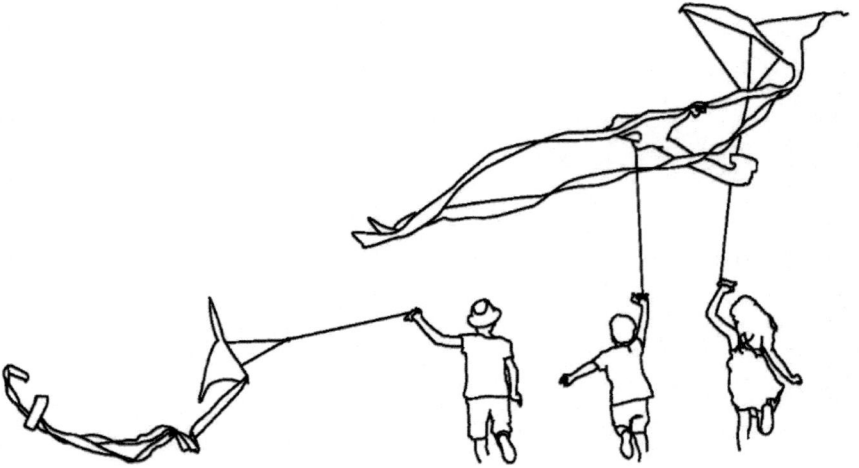

# Foreword

Anne Matthews' wonderful book unpacks and delivers some of the most relevant parenting advice available for new parents or for those of you who are considering becoming parents. One can feel her humility and her wisdom at the same time, and readers experience a sort of privilege as if being nurtured by a loving family aunt.

As a doctor and practitioner, Anne carries the torch of both the mainstream Chiropractic world as well as the less available teachings from the world of the Pre and Perinatal Sciences. I cherish Anne's words. I wish I had this book back when I was a young parent. And now that I am a grandparent, if I had to seek help for my beloved granddaughter, I could think of no one more competent and trustworthy than Anne.

This book will not only help drain the stresses of parenting, but it will also enrich your life in many ways. You will be so glad it accompanied you through your parenting life, especially when your kids are happy, grounded, peaceful, confident and powerful teenagers.

*Karlton Terry*

Author of New Parenting Can Change your World: More Wisdom - Less Stress - Including the Cure for Colic

Website: ktbabytherapy.com

Instagram: kt_baby_therapy

# Introduction

We all share one life experience ... birth. There are many kinds of birth and yet no right birth; it is just the way it is or was, for all the reasons present at the time. Our body and mind remember how it was for us. As we learn to listen to our body and mind, we can help ourselves and in turn teach our babies and children to listen and heed theirs. We can reclaim that authentic, intuitive and self-aware being we were born to be.

In this book, and in sharing stories from parents and children, the progressive guidance tips and tools at the end of each chapter encourage you to practise self-reflection and view the family constellation through the lens of pre and perinatal trauma awareness. We are all on a journey of self-discovery, especially when it comes to having children and helping them work through their challenges, as it gives us as parents a gifted opportunity to revisit and heal our own childhood experiences.

Let's journey together as we learn how to identify underlying pre and perinatal issues from a child's Baby Body Language and how to address them. As we work through some of the issues, reframe our perceptions and re-pattern adaptive behaviours, I encourage you to cultivate a culture of kindness and self-compassion in your life. Offer grace, space, and empathy as you pace the needs of your child and those family members who may initially appear to be resistant to change.

My aim is to navigate a path of listening to both the parents' and child's narratives by using and expanding the repertoire of Baby Body Language tools so the facts will resonate with each family member in a connected way. Or, to put it another way - the issue is in the tissue - the body remembers[1] and that is where you and your child will feel it, sense it and from where we can facilitate change and the re-patterning of thoughts and beliefs. These issues reside in our body's tissues; the joints, muscles, fascial tissue, bones and organs, and they are retold and played out by our mind, our behaviour, our actions and our words. It's not a competition or a blame game with one person being right and the other wrong.

I will share guidance, case study interviews and case study narratives from some of the thousands of parents and children that I have had the privilege to work with over the past 36 years. If you are at a loss to know what the next possible step could be to help your baby or child, my mission is to help you. I trust you will also become empowered to formulate the questions to ask a health or educational professional in pursuing the care of your child and that you will find your voice as their advocate so that both of you can be seen and heard.

One of the first steps for a mum to truly "see and hear" her own baby and child is to intentionally become more present and more aware of her own emotions, thoughts and the feelings in her physical body before and during pregnancy, birth and beyond. In the chapters of this book, you will realise that our family, cultural and societal norms can blind us from intuitively knowing what our baby is telling us.

My approach is to guide parents along a path of understanding with step-by-step problem-solving rather than the traditional reductionist one of reacting to and fixing symptoms. The latter tends to have a longer-term effect of not adequately addressing a child's developmental, physical and emotional issues

---

[1] **Rothschild, Babette. 2000.** The Body Remembers: The Psychophysiology of Trauma and Trauma Treatment. New York: W. W. Norton and Company

which may have negatively impacted their self-confidence and basic life skills. These are often referred to as "the challenges" that the child is currently experiencing.

To offer you more context, I would like to share some of the early influences on my life and vocational journey. In my own family of origin, I am the middle child of a family of seven living children, six girls and one boy. Our eldest sibling, Theresa, my parents' firstborn, died at birth in 1950. Over the years growing up, we more often referred to our family as consisting of seven children rather than eight, which was both the common and expected thing to do at the time. However, our mum, Margaret, would have reminded us in November each year of Theresa's birthday.

The sharing of her birth story, and the unfortunate circumstances surrounding the negative and traumatic birth experience, was always distressing to hear and reflective of the inadequate standard of maternity services in the early years of the National Health Service within the UK. In fact, my dad, Harry did not share his version of the story until 44 years later, prompted by another such loss in our family.

As a teenager and young adult, I was deeply touched by how the triggered emotions of grief and loss did not seem to wane with intensity in the passing years, when Margaret would retell the story with tears in her eyes, even after having given birth multiple times and also having experienced a couple of miscarriages. In sharing her pain, she tried to suppress the depth of her loss in a bid to protect and not overwhelm her daughters with the anguishes of childbirth.

What was also obvious was the various levels of emotional unavailability, within both our immediate and the extended family field, which looked like a reluctance to express emotions;

avoidance of sharing personal details around the pregnancy and the delivery; and a belief system that disregarded birth as a challenge or emotionally traumatic event.

Recognising the lifelong emotional impact of unaddressed issues around birth trauma and loss, together with the lack of emotional support for grieving parents, was also present in many of the families I worked with. I became more aware of the fear, shame, guilt, grief and distrust that contributed to the perpetuation of these unspoken traumas within a family. This situation motivated me to look for answers and help parents and children to navigate the challenges around birth trauma and the connections and beliefs of the family field. This also motivated me to look at how we can interrupt and cut replicating cords of transgenerational traumas and family expectations.

In my early 20s, I read a book by the French obstetrician, Frederick Leboyer - Birth Without Violence[2]. From the title to every page of his poetic verse, coupled with the impactful black and white images of newborns which he used to describe the birth experience from the baby's perspective, this book resonated with me. I recall wondering why, as parents, we would not opt for a non-violent birth for both mum and baby, given the lifelong emotional, psychological and physical impact that can and does occur for both baby and mum.

Unveiling the blind spots in my own perceptions of my extended family dynamics, and the narrative around my parental experiences, has helped me to navigate a path of healing old wounds and traumas, some of which I had unconsciously inherited from my parents and their parents, my ancestors. This path has led

---

[2] Leboyer, F. 1991. Birth Without Violence: The book that revolutionised the way we bring up our children. London: Mandarin Paperbacks

me to a greater understanding of how and why a child can become disconnected from themselves, their siblings and/or their parents.

These questions propelled me along a vocational path involving years of achieving numerous qualifications and immersing myself in deep personal discovery workshops. The challenging soul searching revealed the impacts of my early imprints which saw me suffering the consequences of making challenging life choices and from which I sought a different path.

I discovered that the answers unfold when we are open to learning from, and acknowledging, the stories we have unconsciously created around our very early life experiences in the womb, at birth, after birth and in early childhood. Otherwise, our authentic connection can gradually shift and fragment, moving us towards a disconnected state of being.

Each of us has had a birth experience that has shaped both us and our mums to varying degrees. However, that is not to say that we have all become victims defined by the challenging imprints of the birth experience. In fact, how we relate to and interpret our early birthing experiences, through our nervous system, defines how these early imprints shape the settings of the person we are today. The body keeps the score[3] and that impact on our body shapes how we grow and develop as children into adulthood. All of this can be read, interpreted, validated and addressed, as appropriate, as it is never too late to heal. The good news is that healing can happen naturally, and often without parental interventions, just by the nature of how a child's physical and emotional development evolves. However, there are circumstances in which the healing process gets bogged down and

---

[3] Van der Kolk, B. 2014. The Body Keeps The Score: Mind, Brain and Body in the Transformation of Trauma. Uk. Penguin Books

is expressed by a child's Baby Body Language as unaddressed birth trauma for both mum and baby and in the challenges that a parent recognises their child is experiencing.

Learning to read Baby Body Language will help you make connections that will strengthen your child's natural abilities to heal.

*"Our babies do not come with an instruction manual; we need to learn on the job so let's make the best of this wonderful opportunity!"*

***Anne Matthews***

In my clinical experience, we so often need to go back to the beginning; back to life during pregnancy and our child's birth story and ask the questions, "What happened to you?" and "What happened to me?" rather than the traditional approach of asking, "What is wrong with you?" or "What is wrong with me?"

This book is designed to be read from Chapter One sequentially to the end as the concepts and explanations are sensitively layered to guide you. I offer parents clarity around recognising that an unsettled baby or challenged child often lacks optimal alignment and balance not only physically, but also emotionally, developmentally and physiologically. This would result in the child feeling out of balance and disconnected. Sleep, feeding and bowel issues, hyperactivity, low muscle tone, uncoordinated, developmental delay and persistent crying are some of the tell-tale signs of imbalance and disconnection. Again, these are often considered "challenges", or the child presents as either being challenged or challenging. Some of the therapies and disciplines available in the integrative approach to treating and managing babies and children are discussed in Chapter Six.

In my practice, I aim for a communication style that is non-judgmental, empathetic, and compassionate as I navigate parents to seek a path of being truly present in the moment as they reflect and practise the suggestions made. Being fully present increases one's own self-awareness and helps a parent to have greater empathy in witnessing their child's plight and to recognise their subtle shifts towards self and co-regulation as they respond to treatment.

I introduce the therapeutic power of touch by instructing and guiding parents on basic massage techniques to use with their baby and child to help them release muscle and emotional tension and improve their sensory regulation. As parents become more skilled at massage, they will discover the joy of listening with their hands as they read and connect empathetically with their child.

At the end of each chapter, you will find a section on "Guidance Tips and Tools" which includes self-reflection tips and specific exercises to use with your baby or child at their various developmental stages. In summary, my intention is that this book will help you to:

- gain a greater understanding of how pregnancy shapes birth;
- recognise how the imprints of birth shape your child's development;
- recognise that babies are sensitive and aware through pregnancy, birth, and babyhood;
- empathise with your child from these new perspectives;
- be your child's ally and advocate;
- acknowledge that, as parents, you did what you did in the past with the information that you had at the time;
- as we know better, we do better; and

- accept that regret is the thief of the past and fear the thief of the future.
- As parents we want the very best for our children, so let us begin this journey of discovery and transformation together.

**Anne Matthews**

Belfast, Northern Ireland - October 2023

# Prologue
## What are Early Imprints?

When my younger siblings and I were children, running around after having our bath, my parents would say we were showing off our birth-day suits. As a baby, you were born with your own unique birth-day suit, your coat of many colours. The essence, the sheen and the character of that coat are not only determined by the genes inherited from your parents and from how those first two cells from your parents met - the egg and the sperm at the moment of conception - but also all the experiences and feelings you have had with coming into being. Each living cell in our body has a job to do that was embryologically predetermined when that little fertilised egg travelled along the fallopian tube to implant in your mum's womb and registered to her hormonal system that she was pregnant, and you were discovered.

Before we go any further, I want to reassure you that we all have early imprints and they are not to be considered as a good or bad thing, rather, it is more helpful to consider them as part of what has shaped and moulded us. It is good to know of our early imprints. Your awareness of these early experiences and feelings started at conception as a sense in your soma (body), your physical tissues, and they left their imprints. Then, as you grew and developed inside mum through the first, second and third trimesters, you were aware from the "inside" of her emotions and how she lived her life. You responded and reacted to how her system coped with the everyday ups and downs, the highs and lows, the expectations and the disappointments. These would have left their unique imprints that shaped your developing perception of the world outside the womb.

In the womb, you only perceived the world through your mum; there was no "me", yet. You would have perceived all her emotions, her love, sadness, her grief, anger, her shame, her joy and laughter. You would have become excited, nervous, fearful, happy, disappointed or perhaps a mixture of all these emotions as your birth-day approached.

Together, you actively participated in the initiation and pacing of the contractions of labour and the miraculous uninterrupted journey of a natural vaginal birth, as per your blueprint. You were welcomed and held by your mum in that golden hour, your first hour of life with skin-to-skin contact as you bonded with your mum and crawled to the breast for your first feed.

Although this may not have been your narrative, all your experiences, your imprints, were recorded and hard-wired into your brain and nervous system. These were your original default settings and they laid the foundation for your own unique approach to life and how you live it. These settings were further shaped and layered by the care you received as a newborn and infant, and what supportive relationships and resources were available for your mum in the "fourth trimester", your first year of life. Your actual birth was the beginning of developing a sense of "self" as separate from your mum; the first sense of "me" as a human being in the physical world.

### Making sense of early imprints

Anything that stresses the baby in the womb, during or after birth and in their early years, is referred to as a stressor. For example, smoking and alcohol are now widely accepted as significant stressors during pregnancy and are best avoided. This took decades of education and social change and is still ongoing.

However, there are still numerous other stressors that are not yet regarded as significant, such as the physical, emotional and physiological stressors that can occur during pregnancy and birth. These stressors can cause glitches in the developing brain and nervous system, resulting in an interruption and then delay in the child's development to reach their essential milestones.

When parents of a very anxious teenager seek our help, the teen's early childhood profile helps paint a picture of the baby that their child once was. The perceived "needy" baby can become the oversensitive toddler that experiences separation anxiety when starting nursery school. When they reach the challenges of their teenage years, they may seem to lose their joy and can feel unwell due to anxiety. The interruption from the stressors during pregnancy can impact to some degree on their learning ability, contributing to behavioural issues and their ability for connecting and socialising with parents, family and peers.

I interpret a child's early imprints by reading their body language, posture, gestures and behaviours. Birth imprints can weave mixed threads of memories and experiences from both the present and the past. These threads influence a child's perceptions and beliefs coupled with the narratives from their parents and families and, as a result, the influence stretches back through many generations. Children will have various ways of adapting and surviving experiences that are too overwhelming for them. A child who displays persistent challenging behaviour can often be misunderstood and discounted as just being problematic in the moment rather than full consideration being given to their past. I guide parents in finding a renewed empathy for their child from this PPN perspective as they recognise and acknowledge that the imprints of birth and pregnancy have actually shaped their child.

In later chapters, I will discuss ways to address early imprints and birth trauma which have negatively impacted the nervous systems of babies and young children. We can read and interpret their early imprints and work out where and how to address the patterns of behaviour and movement which have made the child's nervous system (NS) adapt to their new norm.

As parents journey with their child down this parallel path of understanding and acknowledgement, they discover a healing process for both themselves and their children. Often, parents will begin to reflect more on their own early childhood and seek guidance in interpreting the effect of these early life experiences in their adult life - their imprints. This can be a truly transformational journey for many families and one thing that we do know – it is never too late to heal!

# Hello and Welcome to my Treatment Room

In 1988, we formally opened the doors of the Belfast Chiropractic Clinic & Complementary Therapies and since then our Clinic Team have been serving families towards better health and well-being through chiropractic, nutrition, massage, mind coaching, craniosacral therapy and other therapies.

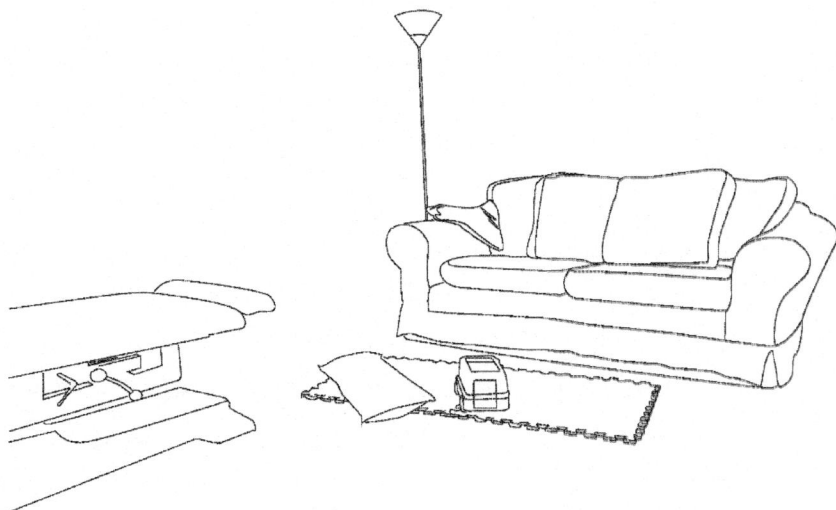

My treatment room is a calm space with light-coloured walls dotted with butterflies and an invitation to just "breathe," displayed above the windows. A mini skeleton looks out from the desk and a slouchy sofa awaits to welcome and wrap around the parents.

Children can find their place in *the nose park*, a fun name I use when inviting a child to lie face down on the treatment bench. Pregnant mummies can also lie face down in the turtle shell and babies are often cosseted in the safety of grown-up arms.

These are the places where our work together can be done. This book, like my room in the clinic, is all of the following:

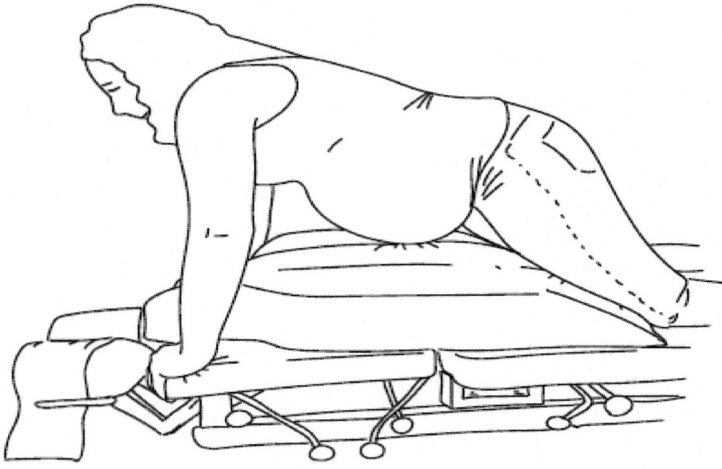

- A safe place; a place for sharing our birth stories and family dynamics; one of facilitation so that the intellectual, physical and emotional parts can become more connected.

- A place where we become more self-aware and other-aware.

- A place of presence and therapeutic calm that allows the body to become aligned and the mind to find connection.

- A place of guidance; tips and tools, finding awareness, understanding, togetherness and play.

- A place of facilitated expansion and growth, where the baby and child can develop, as everyone tunes in at their own pace and as we all get on the same page.

The calming decor reflects this too with clients commenting on how it gives them a sense of reassurance that they will be well cared for. Clients often comment that my presence in the treatment room induces in them a state of relaxation and a readiness to share their stories in confidence and at their own pace. I cultivate this therapeutic presence as I aim to be fully present and connected with those in the room.

This wholesome setting allows me to support and connect with babies, children and their families as I facilitate them in getting into the right relationship and connection with themselves and each other. I educate parents and children on skeletal alignment, joint movement and body balancing within brain development and the neurodevelopmental framework.

My finer touch skills are more chiropractic and craniosacral based, coupled with my empathetic skills of listening and observing which allows me to meet clients' emotional needs as they arise. Expression of emotional issues allows for re-patterning of the body/brain links which paves the way for a greater connection with one's 'felt' sense and a welcome release from old self-limiting patterns.

Throughout this book, I will share case studies and stories, with consent from parents and children from my practice, with the aim of supporting you and your family. These are stories of growth, finding inner connection and self-healing. I will share how I observe babies become more settled, parents become more confident and empowered and children become happier and content in themselves. I see older children progress and improve at school. I see the family dynamics shift as they become more grounded, connected, empathetic and fun-loving. In this book, you may recognise some of the more adaptive behaviours and resonate with the case studies that may feel familiar on several levels.

My mission is to see families become more wholesomely connected both as individuals and as a family unit.

# Chapter One

## Creating a Safe Space

Many babies and young children attend our clinic because they are recognised as being somehow trapped within their bodies and brains with behaviours that are showing *something*. Parents may feel a sense of not knowing what to do next, helpless, worried and fearful. That's okay, this is the place for enquiry and exploration, the place to ask; "What is my child telling me?" Asking for professional support for your child and family is a big step towards the change the family wants to see; almost universally this is for a happier, connected child. The bonus for me is to see a happier and connected family.

Firstly, offering parents an opportunity to complete an intake form before attending their child's first consultation is essential. This is an invitation to detail the concerns they have regarding their child's everyday physical, developmental and emotional needs. They can list the practical challenges around their child, from their pregnancy, birth, and the early days of feeding, sleeping and pooping, to how the child has met or not met their developmental milestones.

Some parents will be very conscientious in ticking the relevant boxes and elaborate on the points in question in the comment sections whereas others will offer a limited amount of background information. Each individual style helps me in gauging and pacing parents right from the beginning so that I can readily meet their emotional needs and expectations.

I will share case studies throughout the book so that you may, in turn, learn from or relate to the families' experiences. Here is the first:

## Raghav - aged four years

At his first consultation, Raghav appeared to me like a child who was totally distracted, as if triggered by a world of inner chaos. He was unable to stand or sit still for more than a few seconds and made quiet groaning-like sounds without words. He struggled to keep his head upright as it lolled about, whilst his eyes rolled back and forth as he tried to focus on me and figure out the treatment room. His parents were corralling the constant movement of his arms and legs and it looked like he would fall over at any moment. There was no let-up.

My recall was that his parents played two different roles in that first session. Mum, Shobba, remained close by her son to protect him from falling or tripping over himself whilst dad, Arjun was keen to engage me in offering him an academic explanation of craniosacral therapy. What was plain and simple from the beginning was that we all needed to get on the same page.

Rather than coming from the perspective of "What's wrong with my child?", I help parents understand the subtle approach of working from the child's perspective and asking the essential questions - "What happened to my child? and "How did they get to this place?"

Before me were two very concerned, devoted and loving parents who explained how they had engaged with many professionals in the past before attending me and both of whom were determined to leave no stone unturned in the search for answers to help their four-year-old son. So, I needed to tune into this unique family dynamic and view things from mum's, dad's and Raghav's perspectives and create a bridge to the therapy on offer.

## A safe space

Providing a safe space for both child and parents, from an energetic point of view, requires building trust and rapport through sensitive questioning and sharing early observations of the situation.

Guiding and pacing parents in this meaningful way resonates with them and reassures them as it stirs their sense of curiosity. This allows parents to find personal space to pause and reflect in terms of both their child's life story and his developmental sequence or steps that may have been interrupted by his early experiences in the womb. It is not about naming and shaming - far from it, this is about reflection and developing a new understanding. Although we cannot change or rewrite history, we initially need to know, and understand, a child's pre and post-birth story to learn from what, and how, they may have experienced it.

## Tell-tale signs of a tough birth

My early observations of Raghav's physical posture and movement prompted a need to invite mum to share her story around her experiences during her pregnancy and his birth. For example, I was curious about the way in which Raghav held his head tilted to one side, the presence of an eye squint, his inability to stand and balance himself evenly on his two feet and the need to prop himself up against a wall to keep upright. His nervous system (NS) appeared so triggered, activated and on edge that he could not keep his arms or legs still. He showed clear physical evidence of having had a tough time being born, of being squashed and compressed. It looked like he was continually searching for his balance point but with no idea as to where it might be. The fact was that Raghav was unable to regulate his nervous system and relied on his parents to help him which they were unwittingly, and yet understandably, doing. Unfortunately, this comes with a price as the child is not really developing their own ability to regulate their nervous system. This is a situation which becomes a greater uphill battle for parents as the child gets older and develops more compensatory strategies.

Raghav had been a long-awaited baby. Shobba's pregnancy coincided with a very busy and intense period at work which involved spending long hours on her feet in the laboratory as a scientist in London. She had experienced some back and leg pain. During her second trimester, her father became terminally ill and she travelled to India to be with him. On her return to the UK, her father died suddenly and she immediately took another long-haul flight to be with her mum for her father's funeral. Shobba returned to London in a state of grief only to learn that her husband Arjun's mum had taken seriously ill too and her father's brother had died unexpectedly. The third trimester included a period of deep grief, mourning and sadness.

Shobba described a long labour resulting in a forceps delivery and Raghav being an unsettled newborn. The family moved from London to Northern Ireland when Raghav was around three months old and, shortly afterwards, his paternal grandmother died. The family had also been victims of a house burglary before moving. Shobba recognised that there was a lot of unexpected and unwanted stress during her pregnancy and for her newborn, which would not have been ideal for Raghav but, equally, she reflected that was just how life was at the time and she did her best to manage her situation. It was Raghav's parents' opinion that the MMR vaccination "knocked him for six." Arjun responded to their situation by focusing a lot of his time on researching help for Raghav together with managing the family business.

Shobba's narrative of her pregnancy and birth experiences would suggest that she probably had high levels of stress hormones within her system during these most trying times. She also described the bond and loving connection she had with her parents and the need to travel to them given her father's terminal illness and, later, sad demise.

There was probably a physical constriction issue for baby Raghav in the womb too, given the history of his mum's back and leg pain which she mentioned had started in the second trimester. Such symptoms are often indicative of a mechanical restriction and imbalance within the dynamics of the mum's pelvic joints, muscles and ligaments, all of which support the baby in her pelvic basket. If that were the case, the baby may have been positioned off-centre in the womb resulting in less space for them to move around and practise their primitive reflexes (or foetal movement exercises) in preparation for delivery and birth. The reasons for a long labour could also be due to the quality and productivity of the contractions which may not have been optimal in moving the baby down, into and through the birth canal.

In fact, if a woman in labour is required to lie on her back, the active participation of her physical body in the delivery process is restricted as she would not be benefiting from the assistance of gravity compared to if she were in an upright position. Also, lying on the back restricts the movement of the sacrum (the tailbone area) which is a vital bone at the back of the pelvis that the baby within can be pushed up against by the contractions during the descent into the birth canal. The baby will often get stuck here and be unable to move further down into the canal. When a mum is in a more upright position during labour, she has more space in her pelvis for her baby and she can readily adjust her position to facilitate the passing of the baby's head and face against the inner side of the sacrum as she senses the baby move past the sacrum and descend down through the birth canal. The illustration below shows optimal alignment of the baby in the womb.

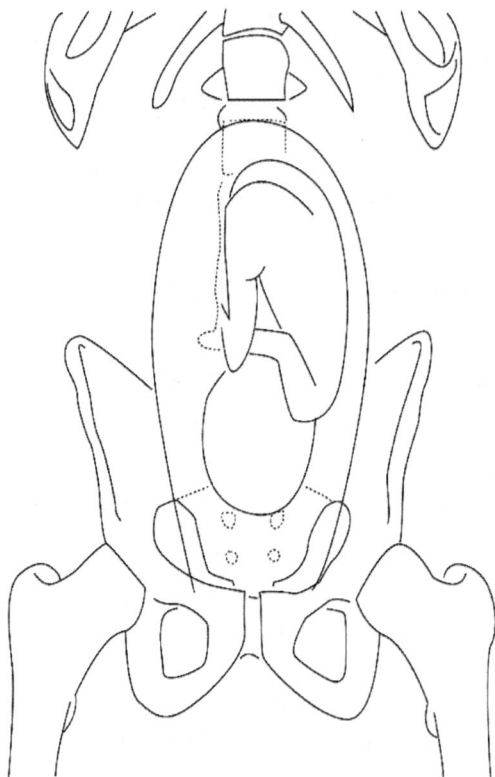

When there is a misalignment issue, resulting in the baby's head and shoulders being compressed and stuck in the birth canal, physical assistance and intervention from the medical team are often required. This feeling of 'stuckness' by the baby will also be interpreted by a birthing mum as having intense and unbearable labour pain in her lower back due to the baby's head being forced up against and dragged by the mum's sacral plexus; a rich bed of nerves at the bottom of the spine.

To relieve this situation, in Raghav's case, involved the spoons of the forceps being placed on either side of his head whilst inside mum.

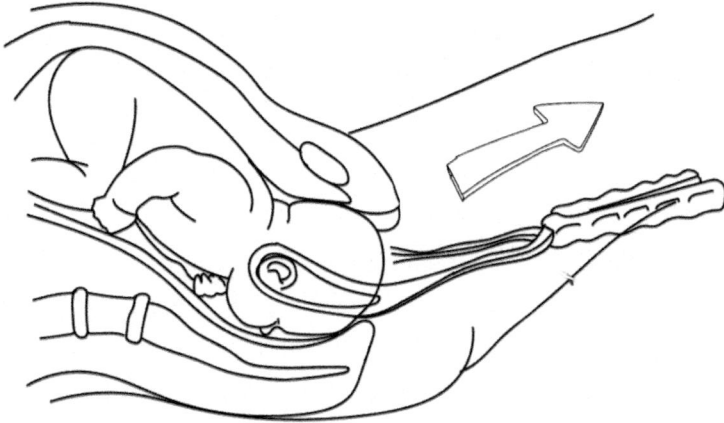

Such a delivery by forceps involves a gentle pulling and rotational downward, tugging movement to deliver the baby safely. As every action and intervention has consequences, a forceps delivery can leave an imprint in the baby's body and nervous system. For example, a birthing baby may instinctively recoil against the tug and pressure of the unexpected forceps. Such a response is recorded in a baby's nervous system and can trigger shock and fear which would leave an imprint in his system. Such newborns can be observed as having a rapid and shallow breathing pattern, a hypersensitivity to touch, as in handling the baby, and a sensitivity to loud mechanical sounds.

As seen in the illustration overleaf, a newborn delivered by forceps might also have pressure marks on their face, a noticeable head tilt to one side and a twist in their body which is usually more obvious to a parent when the baby is lying on their back or when propped up sitting in a car seat, for example. Mums will often describe such a baby as having a short and tight neck which is difficult to access to dry after a bath. The baby's head and neck have effectively been pulled back and down into their shoulders.

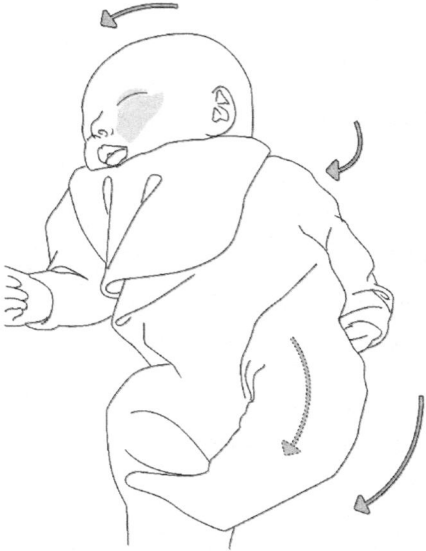

This postural pattern can be seen in older babies or toddlers who hold their shoulders raised tightly and, when brought to mum's attention, she will comment on how the child gets distressed when having their clothes put on or off over their head. Such babies can be easily startled, or become resistant and cry readily when a parent tries to direct their arms into the sleeves of a top. A newborn with a head tilt may appear to be fussy on feeding at the breast or on one particular side. This is because turning their head to the side or lying on one side is uncomfortable for them.

By voicing these observations of the necessary adaptations of the baby or child, mums then become more confident about sharing the practical things that they have noticed in the activities of daily living, such as putting the baby's arms into sleeves and changing the baby's nappy (or diaper) which upsets the baby.

These difficulties are the challenges that mum has known intuitively about her baby but was unable to express or understand until a possible cause and effect was explained practically in this way and things suddenly make a whole lot of sense to the parents. This is how we get on the "same page" of understanding and becoming more aware of what babies might have experienced in their journey during pregnancy and at birth and how they have adapted to the physical and emotional imprints which have remained with them.

Raghav was that very baby - difficult to breastfeed, to dress, undress and to settle. He was not comfortable being handled or put down to settle for sleep, no matter how super careful his parents were, as his nervous system had been set or calibrated to high alert, more than likely from the shock he experienced around his delivery and birth following an already highly stressful pregnancy. It was like an accumulation of stressors one on top of the other which then dictated how his NS reacted to the next perceived stressful event. It's possible that the misalignment of his head and neck on his shoulders together with the muscular tension that he was holding throughout his spine and pelvis were related to his delivery. Namely, the compression on either side of his head from the clenching of the forceps blades and the tugging on his neck as he was pulled out of the birth canal.

It's helpful for parents to understand that a safe delivery at birth may have had an impact on their baby and leave a physical and emotional imprint. Compression from the forceps spoons can contribute to bony restrictions around where the cranial bones of the skull connect to each other (cranial sutures); for example, around the ears at the sides of the baby's head, into the jaw joints and deep inside the skull where the cranial bones interconnect behind the eyes' sockets. The consequence of this necessary, often lifesaving, medical intervention can contribute to the misalignment of the position of the eyes. This means that the muscles controlling the eyes are not balanced which may result in a baby having a squint. When a baby experiences this type of birth, we understand that it is perceived as an intense physical and emotional experience that is recorded in the baby's brain and NS, his unique original settings. Remember, the body keeps the score.[4] Such an experience will leave the baby or child feeling constantly on the alert as they tend to be startled and cry readily at unexpected loud noises, bright lights or abrupt handling.

A toddler or older child who has experienced a forceps delivery birth can often display behaviour patterns of not wanting to be rushed or pushed into situations, often noticeable when dressing or being put into their car seat. Such children can also be very sensitive when their head or neck is being touched, for example, when having their hair shampooed, brushed, having a haircut or when a hat is pulled onto their head.

In my clinical experience, the challenges of an older child with a similar birth story may be seen as being very sensitive to criticism, when being told "no" or when not able to get their own way around straightforward everyday activities of family life. They can also tend to be wakeful children as they are unable to remain asleep when lying flat on their backs. This is witnessed by the over-tired and frustrated parent who settles their baby by cradling them to sleep in their arms, only for the baby to then wake up abruptly when being transferred to lie in their cot. Some parents may misread this situation as the baby becoming spoiled and wanting only to fall asleep in their parents' arms or, perhaps, they think that the baby has developed a dislike for their cot or room, for example.

[4] Van der Kolk, B. 2014. The Body Keeps The Score: Mind, Brain and Body in the Transformation of Trauma. Uk. Penguin Books

However, so often the unsettled baby of this nature is simply unable to let go of the fixed tension in the joints and muscles that keep their neck and head upright, forward and tilted. These physical restrictions also make the child feel anxious, always on the alert and in need of support, comfort and the reassuring embrace of a parent in order to settle and regulate their nervous system.

Interestingly, when a birth experience is far too intense and overwhelming for a baby's nervous system, the baby may adapt to protect themselves by effectively appearing to shut down their nervous system. As a result, the baby may appear not to move or cry in response to situations which would startle other babies. These children can develop adaptive strategies that mean they tune out or switch off from situations which they perceive may cause them undue stress. The baby learns to dissociate from the experience as their nervous system protects them and they feel safer. Babies like this are often described as "a good baby that doesn't cry" or "a lazy baby" that is content to sit and does not appear to be curious or inquisitive to explore their surroundings.

However, the reality is that some babies and young children have been deeply shocked by their early experiences during pregnancy and birth, leaving imprints on their nervous system. This theme around these early imprints and understanding a child's resulting behaviour and adaptive strategies will be developed as other stories are shared in future chapters.

### What is my baby telling me?

Many parents of young babies will often comment, "If only I could understand what he is telling me." The fact is babies are telling us things *all the time;* we parents just need to learn to read the cues and understand what they are sharing and communicating with their BBL movements and gestures. A common myth is that babies are not much fun to be with until six months old when they can start to interact with their parents. The belief that a baby is uncommunicative until they start sitting up, interacting and using early sounds and words is far from the truth. Babies are expressing their needs in the sounds that they make, in their body movements, breathing pattern and in the eye contact they have (or don't have) with a parent. On some level, I suspect that many parents do have an inkling of this. Parents often have a hidden "knowing" that they don't quite trust. Furthermore, the myths and stories that are spun and retold within the extended family and friendship groups around children's development and expectations tend to make parents doubt the validity of their own intuitiveness.

Nowadays, there seems to be an over-reliance on online child development apps that inform parents of what to expect at the next growth spurt, developmental or regression stage. In my opinion, these can distract parents from connecting through the joy of discovering, with awe and wonderment, how their baby and child reveals and shares their developmental steps with them; or worse, the parent who feels disappointed and ashamed that their child is not achieving the perceived gold standard as per the App. Encouraging parents to tune into their own intuitive observations of their child, and *then* use external material as a backup, can be very empowering and a great confidence builder in positive, conscious and empathetic parenting.

A baby will persist in letting parents know that they want their needs met, for example, by insistent crying and wakefulness. With guidance, parents start to get a sense, like a dawning, that their baby is trying to tell them something.

Parents often seek out my help as a last resort and, on meeting the baby or child, I inwardly and silently congratulate the child on persisting with their parents! The journey towards change and transformation for the family has just begun. Most parents tend not to be disconnected or narcissistic in how they interact with their children, but some can be. It is important for new parents to acknowledge that they are products of their own babyhood and childhood in terms of whether their emotional and physical needs were heard, met and attended to adequately. Although we may tend to repeat history in how we parent and communicate with our children, this can also be an ideal opportunity for parents to respond and interact differently to the early experiences that they had. Parents who invest time in reflection and connection, as they learn and engage with the BBL tools and practise being in the present moment for their baby and child, will reap the rewards as their children grow and develop into teenagers and caring young adults.

However, parents can be totally unaware that their own early, unaddressed childhood issues are being triggered by their baby. When those parental childhood issues are being triggered, parents may seem to not agree with their partner on how best to attend to their baby's needs and will often fall foul of the common myths that you can spoil a baby by co-sleeping, feeding on demand, lifting and cuddling them rather than letting them cry it out. It is extremely insightful for parents to spend time together focussing on gently developing such conversations and teasing out the myths of their own respective early extended family dynamics.

The reality is that we need to give our babies a voice from deep inside the womb. Reading and interpreting BBL is a way parents are facilitated to stop, sense into the moment and open themselves to what their baby wants to share with them.

Listening to the mum's narrative, as the baby's advocate, whilst tracking the baby's movements and agitation levels, or active BBL, can be extremely revealing. Hearing the pre and post-birth story, from both mum's and baby's perspectives, is further helped as I listen to dad's side of the birth story and is both very rewarding and revealing to the baby and parents. Remember, babies can be very forgiving when they realise we are trying to communicate on their level. Reflect on the fact that it's never too late to address a birth and childhood issue.

**Helping Raghav to reorient his skewed Nervous System(NS)**

That first session was the start of a journey that would see Raghav respond positively to his treatment programme and guided management from his keen and committed parents, as we will see later in this chapter. As Raghav responded, his NS became more regulated as he was able to reorientate his midline awareness and sense of balance. This, in turn, allowed him to progress through many missed vital developmental steps to achieve more of his age-appropriate milestones.

It was a journey of becoming more communicative, more coordinated and physically active and more emotionally aware. As he caught up on his delayed development, he gradually became more sociable and started to both acknowledge and play with other children at school. Observing this family become more wholesomely connected, as Raghav's brain and NS become more integrated, was an absolute pleasure to behold.

However, Raghav's parents initially attended me with a belief that Raghav's behavioural and developmental issues needed fixing. On one hand, this was understandable. However, the concept of "fixing a child" is an over-simplistic viewpoint that is prevalent within our healthcare system and tends to be dismissive of what may have happened to that child in their early pre-birth, birth and post-birth experiences. Like so many parents, including myself at one time, Raghav's parents sought out many different types of therapy and medical opinions in their endeavours to "fix" Raghav. The repeated disappointments from the random approach offered by professionals in the health system, together with a lack of sustained progress in their pursuits around nutrition, occupational therapy and physiotherapy, was resulting in the parents being distracted and at odds with each other. It was as if they were on a non-stop treadmill working in parallel with each other to find solutions. They had very little time for personal connection within the family as they were dedicating hours to researching exercise programmes and preparing wholly organic-based cooked meals from scratch.

Let me reassure you that the above therapies and nutrition support are extremely important, but these valuable opportunities are often wasted and left by the wayside because they are not offered in a sequential bespoke manner to meet the child's individual needs.

The first step is to identify the early interrupted stages of development so that the child's nervous system can be adequately supported - then the child will tend to be more receptive to what these disciplines and lifestyle changes have to offer. Raghav's NS was just not sufficiently ready for these individual disciplines to make a significant difference.

If this resonates with you, or you too have tried every type of breast and bottle feeding, nutritional regimes, medical treatments, therapies and exercise programmes, then do continue reading about what worked well for Raghav and his family.

## Helping Raghav to feel safe in his own skin

Facilitating Raghav to feel safe in his own skin was paramount as his early nervous system settings were set on high alert, fight, flight and disconnect mode. These are much-needed adaptations that a child's system resorts to for the child's mortal survival (which is not an exaggeration!). From Raghav's perspective, however, he would have probably felt like his body was constantly about to fall over and as if his head was bobbing on his neck precariously, which is a scary state for a young child to be experiencing.

Children like Raghav need help in developing a healthy awareness and self-control over different parts of their body and learning to relate to them. He needed to develop an awareness of where his legs, arms, hands and feet were at any one time in relation to his midline so that his core balance could develop. Developing his core balance would then allow him to stand upright, feel balanced and more coordinated.

It was also necessary to gently release the physical tensions and restriction patterns that held parts of his body and head. A child readily improves and develops a connection with their midline, in both their upper and lower body, through the tandem efforts to develop their core balance and release tensions held in the body. This is necessary for developing coordination and both sensory and spatial awareness. As a child feels safe and more confident in their physical body, their brain and nervous system start working together in harmony and they develop the ability to self-regulate more effectively. The child then becomes more physically able, more emotionally confident and more willing to try new things that help him to grow up more easily and readily. Such children will develop a greater sense of self-motivation, use their initiative and present as feeling happier.

# The Power of Touch

Raghav's parents were advised on basic massage techniques to relieve his discomfort and to give him sensory reassurance. Massage helped him to become more aware of his arms, legs, back, shoulders and head so that he could feel more connected, balanced and grounded within his body. The language of sense and touch is developed very early on in pregnancy and well in advance of verbal language; it is how a mum and baby connect in the womb. The baby within is aware of mum's fluctuating emotions from joy, happiness, tiredness, grief, and hunger to sadness and fear as he learns how she expresses and responds to those feelings. The baby is aware of how mum strokes and touches her body and caresses her baby bump and how dad or partner caresses, hugs and supports mum and their baby within her. The baby in the womb is also very aware when this is not the case and there are negative emotions and disconnects in the inter-relational family field in that early family dynamic.

Most parents understand the importance of early skin-to-skin contact for babies and recognise that it not only calms the baby but also that it is very empowering, reassuring and rewarding for the parent. There is a touch hunger in young babies and from touch comes important developmental stimulation which includes a sense of the baby discovering their own body. A young baby will become more aware of their midline, the front and back of their body, and the left and right of their midline as they roll from side to side and onto their tummy and then onto their back. At the same time, babies are gradually discovering their mouth and lips with their fingers and hands as they practise sucking, gnawing and later chewing, biting and eating. In Raghav's case, he missed out on exploring the natural sequence of these early developmental stages which, in turn, interrupted his natural sequence of the individual stages as his nervous system was preoccupied with simply surviving. It was time for a second chance at meeting his developmental milestones.

---

*"The first classroom is in a mother's womb."*
**Eric Adams**

---

The art of touching through a sequence of massage techniques is such a useful tool for parents. Massage is very effective for a child who is not able to stay still, has recurrent wakefulness, has lack of meaningful eye contact, is unable to follow instructions and is not appearing to listen. All these adaptive behaviours would have been holding the child back from progressing developmentally to the degree that they were not feeling safe, confident and reassured in their own body.

As parents embrace a daily massage routine for their child, with conscious intention, compassion and love, they witness how their child can move into a place of ease and calm. They see their child feeling more safe, more embodied and self-aware as they become more connected with themselves and the earth. Parents observe their child starting to regulate their own nervous system and develop new, balanced behavioural patterns as they move away from their old adaptations. It sets the scene for a child to become more aware of the endeavours of their caregivers and others, which enables spontaneous loving and appreciative interactions as the child breaks away from the old fear, fight, flight and freeze-inducing behaviour patterns.

As parents work together with their BBL-aware practitioner, by improving their massage and other skills, they begin to experience awe and wonderment as they discover the changes in their child and the positive knock-on effect within the family. Parents feel more empowered and more settled within their own nervous system from a sense of achievement and the much-needed signs of hope on the horizon. This also helps parents to become more curious and receptive to the tasks that they are set to do with their child and whets their appetite for more of the same. Actions are often louder than words!

### Pacing parents

Pacing parents and their child is important, both in the individual session and within a series of sessions. Initially, when parents attend, they often come with an expectation and hope that drifts back into the mindset that there is going to be a "quick fix" for their child at every level.

A child, on the other hand, may have an expectation to the contrary and expect that somehow, as the therapist, I will broker a situation where their parents can hear and understand them and realise that they are not in need of fixing. This can create a potential loyalty conflict between how the practitioner interacts and moves forward with the parents and, separately, with the child. Before we can progress in a session, there needs to be an understanding and energetic connection between mum and child. In summary, one needs to facilitate a starting point for establishing awareness, recognition and acknowledgement of the past trauma and the negative effect that it had on the child's emotional and physical development and the negative impact on mum. This is not just the child's issue and often it is the mum and dad that need to be guided and educated to develop their receptivity to the child's perspective. This approach ensures that we are all singing from the same hymn sheet so that we can successfully continue. We will wonder aloud together, with parents and child, and simply extend our curiosity and compassion so they need not hold their stories on their own, within their bodies, or repress their emotions. Rather, we may now come to understand the extent and depth of their emotions. Although babies and toddlers may not have the words, they are trying to show and express their feelings, frustrations, and dis-ease (or distress) in other ways through their BBL.

Ongoing checking in, looping back and reviewing progress with a mum and dad in the session is necessary to make sure we are all connected and have the same understanding. This technique helps parents to understand that the aim of treatment is to help their child to regulate his nervous system at the point he is at, at that moment in time. However, as a child and parents may not be on the same page then the juggle is to deal with the person whose nervous system needs most urgent regulation to move to the next stage. Interestingly, that person is not always the child.

For example, in a session, a mum may suddenly feel some guilt or denial around the experience that her baby may have had at his challenging birth. Here, the tricky part is to facilitate a shift so that a mum can sense into her baby's experience and acknowledge that it was tough for them too. There is no fault here, nor is it being attributed, but a baby does want a mum (and dad) to acknowledge their specific experience during birth, their birth trauma, and help them move on from the negative experience as they integrate it into their nervous system.

My approach can take various strands, from simply demonstrating and facilitating a change of emotions and feelings within the body, within one moment in time, to more factual explanations of child neurodevelopment. The first is referred to as somato emotional releasing and can be facilitated in each family member, either separately or together. As a truly transformational and healing experience process, it improves, builds and strengthens the bonding, attachment and connection between mum and baby, and with both parents. The aim is to assist a child to move forward from their stuck, defensive patterns and adaptive behaviours as they release their suppressed emotions and develop the understanding that, although these had been adaptive and helpful on a basic survival level at the time, they are no longer appropriate and are, in fact, detrimental in holding the child back from expanding into new developmental horizons.

### Guiding Raghav's parents

Much of my work in the first and subsequent sessions is in observing the child and listening to the family story. Gentle inquiry of the more challenging pieces of their narrative is important. Parents who have a highly vigilant child whose nervous system is on high alert, resulting in the child continuously moving, will often mention how they could not imagine that their child would remain still long enough to have any bodywork done on them. This is another myth that gets busted in my room.

In his initial session, ongoing tracking of Raghav's BBL cues, whilst his parents settled into the engagement of the initial consultation and explanation of my treatment approach, facilitated his readiness and trust for doing bodywork with him. Parents will often witness this as their child gravitates energetically towards me when the timing is right for body work treatment to begin.

Contrary to expectations, it is not a case of chasing a child around the room or pinning them to a bench to offer and deliver their treatment. In fact, Raghav moved towards me and pushed his back and legs against my knees as I sat in my inviting comfy tub chair waiting for him to decide when he wanted to engage with me.

I showed him the tube of massage cream and spoke softly in a way which sought his permission as I explained where and how I was planning to massage him. Children may not fully understand exactly what is being said but they certainly understand my intention.

Raghav simply welcomed me in as he moved closer to sit awkwardly on my lap. I gently but firmly massaged his low back muscles, just below and above his waistline, and across his shoulder girdles and neck under his loose-fitting t-shirt. Generally, it is not necessary to undress a child in this situation as that can be too overwhelming for them which can subsequently trigger their NS negatively and they would then recoil and pull away.

Making a soft audible breath by rhythmically inhaling and exhaling, whilst simultaneously massaging and stretching Raghav's trigger points in his muscles, directed him to copy me as he became more sensory aware. As he tuned into my breathing rhythm, he visibly calmed and wriggled more closely to me for a minute or so before reflexively pulling away into his old defensive recoil pattern of movement and then returned to me again to repeat the process. By pacing his needs, and giving him some slack to pull away from me whilst remaining in physical contact with him, he settled into the hands-on treatment. Throughout, I kept him safely contained in an imaginary ring that surrounded my chair, which was positioned directly and closely in front of his parents sitting on the settee, who looked on in relief and awe.

As Raghav's NS settled, I was able to release the restricted joints and an area of muscle tension that he had at the base of his neck and across his shoulders which allowed him to relax as the soft tissues softened. He slowly fell asleep in my arms as I continued to work on his head using craniosacral techniques of gentle touching and releasing of the impacted cranial sutures.

His parents were also invited to become aware of their breathing rhythm and to actively practise breathing in slowly from the belly for the count of four and exhaling fully for the count of eight. This is known as vagal breathing[5] as it stimulates the vagal nerves and relieves stress. As parents, we often mirror the tension and stress that our child is holding and, equally, this can be reversed when a child copies and mirrors their parents' level of nervous tension. It is important for parents, as the adults, to take responsibility and to become actively aware of the level of tension that they may be holding in their body and to consciously practise releasing it.

Common postural tension patterns, which parents are often unaware of in themselves, involve holding their breath for short periods of time whilst keeping the shoulders raised in a stressed protective pattern. Parents are encouraged to practise postural and breath self-awareness when massaging their child at home. These are invaluable techniques to stimulate the part of the nervous system, the parasympathetic NS, which calms the body back down. Mum and dad texted me after their first session to share that their son, who they had mentioned rarely settled on car journeys or for sleep, had slept the entirety of the one-hour journey back home.

The priority before our second session was for Shobba and Arjun to practise and complete Raghav's nightly massage, focus on their own individual feelings of reflection and connection and facilitate their child to walk and be outdoors as much as possible. It was heart-warming to learn of the immediate progress in

---

[5] Vagal breathing involves the practice of deep, slow, repetitive breathing that stimulates the vagus nerve which serves as the body's super-highway, carrying information between the brain and the internal organs to control the body's response in times of rest and relaxation by lowering the heart rate, among other physiological changes.

Raghav's verbal communication skills, together with a flourishing interest in his classmates, as his physical coordination and balance progressed day by day. Shobba and Arjun can take full credit for this through their well-intentioned parenting, self-reflection, willingness and dedication to learning new ways in how to support their son. Consequently, Raghav responded at every step of the way, growing in both physical and emotional confidence. His own sense of fun, humour and adventure blossomed as his parents were encouraged to nurture an "I can do" mentality.

Such a healthy and wholesome transformation is only possible when a child's brain and nervous system are facilitated to transition out of the protective fight/flight and dissociated modes to the more balanced, coordinated and integrated modes involving physical movement and social engagement. This allows a child to be more receptive to the delights of progressing in physical activity and play, love of nature, recognition of and communication with others, independent dressing, feeding and self-care together with having empathy for family and friends.

It is of paramount importance that the BBL practitioner facilitates and paces the parents and child to review and re-evaluate before each session. This ensures that everyone within the family field optimises connection, and safe containment and operates from a calmer pace to provide a place of safety, growth and development.

### The Parents' Story

*"When pregnant with Raghav, I spent two months in India with my parents due to my father's ill health and was still deeply grieving my father's death when Raghav was born, after a very long labour. Within just a few weeks, my mum-in-law also died and so our household was one of both joy and mourning.*

As Raghav wasn't meeting his developmental milestones, we were availing of, and searching out, different types of treatment programmes. We were referred to Anne Matthews by another chiropractor who recommended her as an experienced paediatric practitioner with a penchant for working with children who had developmental challenges," said dad Arjun. "Meeting Anne was a relief. If I am honest, we had been absorbing so much information from so many sources, which we were willing to learn about, but equally, we wanted to know what the right path was and if we were on it! There are four things that Anne's approach and techniques helped us with right away, that we hadn't experienced before:

- We were able to drop our feelings of guilt around Raghav's pregnancy and birth.

- We learned, through Anne, to work in real time on what our child's BBL was showing us at any particular moment.

- We found our voice and were able to express ourselves. Parents benefit from being listened to by a professional.

- We had someone that we could ask any of our questions of and who gave us step-by-step guidance from session to session.

"After the very first treatment of body work and craniosacral therapy, Raghav slept for the one-hour drive back home and started to sleep well at night from that session on. Day by day, we watched our son unfold into a completely different child."

Shobba tells us more about that unfolding.

"One of our daily routines has become a trip to the local forest park. At first, Raghav walked and ran very haphazardly, with his head off to one side. Within 24 hours of his first session, he was running with his head straight. We watched as he grew more confident after each session and found that our confidence in him grew too.

"As parents, we want to talk about the dramatic changes in our son; first, he started running and no longer waddled, then he wanted to try out new things, like exploring in the park. He then tried new things on his own such as the climbing frame. It made us smile and we felt excited for him. We were guided to allow Raghav to practise his developmental stages from rolling to creeping to crawling as we came to understand and read the cues of his Baby Body Language. We realised he was not ready to do things that were out of sequence. Instead, we guided and allowed him first to climb the stairs by crawling up, then to go up and down the stairs unaided, walk backwards and then watched with amazement as he climbed the stairs one after the other, without holding onto the rail.

"After his third session of this combination of body work and craniosacral therapy, it appeared as if a surge of energy was released and he became more connected and engaging. We were taught by Anne to let Raghav take the lead and do things at his own pace as that would help give our child the confidence to take the lead and initiative in everything that he does. As his physical confidence improved so did his use of language - one word at a time," said Arjun. "Our daily time at the park is our father and son bonding opportunity to enjoy the beauty of nature and is also occupational therapy for him as he uses the playground equipment, including the climbing frame and plank. We massaged him daily to Anne's instructions and his body quickly responded in that he lost all his past fears. Previously, he would not walk on grass or stony surfaces whereas now he is both agile and flexible and skips along. He is also good at making his needs known which has removed a lot of the frustration that we were experiencing, and we are looking forward to seeing how his interests will develop.

*"Anne and the information that she shared with us on reading BBL has worked a miracle. As a mum, I feel so lucky to have had her guidance and I want to share these particular gems with the reader.*

- *As a parent you must be able to look after yourself emotionally to be able to look after your child.*

- *Go at your child's pace. Let them try and do things at their pace and just be there with only a little support.*

- *Do the nightly massage routine to ease their tight muscles as it calms both the child and parents.*

- *Offer your child lots of outdoor physical play and sensory exposure to nature.*

*"It is wonderful to see our child, at five years old, accepted by his classroom peers and his emerging "Jack-the-lad" personality. He understands everything that is said to him and has a sparkle in his eyes that he just did not have before. After just 12 months of sessions, his words had greatly increased – including the words for cake and biscuit! We started to sing nursery rhymes all day long.*

*"The tips and tools that we gathered as we progressed through Anne's programme have motivated us as parents to keep trying and to be creative with our child as we observed the immediate benefits of treatment; Raghav got taller and straighter, more flexible, co-ordinated and now walks with his head upright and looking forward. This is a complete contrast to how he used to just sit in the corner and fiddle with the sensory toys we gave him. Now he loves to run, climb and seek out a thrill on any equipment he hasn't used before.*

*"Through understanding Raghav's BBL, we have learned that there are lots of options, possibilities and solutions. It made sense to us that a child has a natural developmental sequence in achieving their milestones and that every child will meet these in a*

*specific order, in one way or another, if they are provided with the right tools and opportunities to do so."*

## Shobba's and Arjun's Mantra for Success

*"Anne positively empowers parents with knowledge and gave us both hope and focus to help Raghav develop an 'I Can Do It' attitude. It has become our mantra. It was clear to us that Raghav understood straight away that Anne would be good for him and was there to help him on his journey. We celebrate every achievement and say thank you for it. We have learned to focus on the solution through using our backpack of guidance tips and tools and we know that Anne is equipping Raghav with his."*

## In Summary

For parents of a baby who is having difficulty sleeping, eating or settling; or a child who is struggling with school and making friends; or who has been given a diagnosis involving a developmental issue, I encourage you to reflect on their early life experiences in the womb, at birth and as a newborn. Such reflection will help you recognise the impact of early imprints and is the first step in finding a solution. An intense and challenging birth can be difficult to navigate and often leaves both physical and emotional stress patterns within the baby, mum and the family. Focussing on building confidence through connection reinforces that you, as parents, can learn to meet the needs of your baby and child.

My mission is to help parents relate to their baby or child's early experiences in an empathetic and informative way, by equipping them with the knowledge, understanding and tools to become more connected and authentic in their bonding and attachment.

As all parents tend to benefit from some guidance, we will end each chapter of this book by sharing with you a set of guidance tips and tools to equip your parenting backpack of useful resources. There is also a reflective exercise to support you in fully integrating the learning that each chapter has revealed.

Guidance
Pack

Tips &
Tools

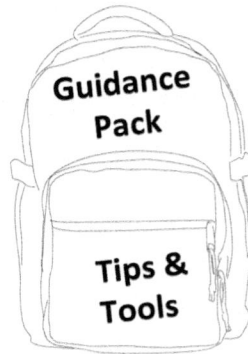

*"Focus on your breathing rhythm to help you monitor your emotions."*

**Awareness**

**Six steps in creating an energetic "safe" space for your child:**

- Pause and note what you are feeling at the first signs of being triggered by your child's behaviour.

- As you pause, sense and name the emotion you are feeling.

- Breathe into the emotion (count 1, 2, 3, 4) then breathe it out (count 1, 2, 3, 4, 5, 6, 7, 8), as if you're breathing it down your body, into your legs then your feet and out into the ground. Repeat. Repeat this 1:2 vagal breathing practice regularly.

- Use the pausing and the sensing of your self-awareness to buy time to respond as you become more grounded rather than impulsively reacting to your child.

- In the moment, see, hear and read your child's needs and emotions to help them feel seen and heard so they can shift towards feeling safe as they regulate their own NS.

- Practising the delicate art of responding rather than reacting helps you to connect in the moment with your child.

**Six steps to help your child become more self-aware:**

- Massage your child regularly to help them become more aware of their body and emotions.

- Notice your child's breathing pattern as they release tension during and after a massage.

- Offer your child opportunities to stretch and play outdoors daily.

- Use fun rhymes, songs and dance movements to help your child discover and be more aware of their limbs, head, face and torso.

- Add adventure walks, play, climbing, crawling, bike riding and jumping on a trampoline to their day.

- Recognise, praise and be in awe of their achievements, no matter how small!

## Reflections

**Six steps to help you reflect on your own feelings, emotions and behaviours, please consider the next four questions in your heart before answering:**

- How are you feeling just now?

- Where do you feel those emotions in your body?

- How do you think your child is feeling?

- Where do you think they hold their tensions in their body?

- Trust your intuition - don't worry, you'll get more practice as you read through the book.

- With each chapter, record your thoughts and feelings in your journal and watch as the answers to your questions unfold.

# Chapter Two

## Pacing a Child and their Parents

Appreciating the need to have clear and recognisable behavioural boundaries is essential for every member of a family. It also helps them in other relationships external to the family, for example, when a child is settling into daycare or school. The subtle establishment of such boundaries may not be immediately obvious to some parents as they may be unaware of the early tell-tale signs of not being in tune in their relationship with their baby. For example, reflect on the case of a mum whose child has had a series of ongoing medical challenges since birth. This mum may tend to overcompensate selflessly when attending to every need of the baby. Such a mum may be driven by an underlying feeling of guilt, as she perceives her child has been a victim of the circumstances of his birth, to the extent that this mum will tend to put his needs and wants before many of her own. The child who is familiar with such attention may have also developed adaptive strategies in response to having all his needs met whereupon he will expect his mum to give greater priority in attending to his needs regardless of hers. From an outsider's point of view, this trait could be interpreted as the child having become more needy, demanding and controlling with age, for example. Such a child could be regarded as lacking value, compassion and respect in regard to his relationship with his mum and other family members.

Establishing subtle behavioural and emotional boundaries starts very early, as early as in the womb, and then progressively in babyhood. The boundaries are developed as a mum attends to her baby's basic needs with compassionate, loving care and attention as she responds to the cues from reading and interpreting his unique BBL together with recognising and considering her own emotional needs. An adequate family support system needs to surround a new mum. This is well documented in the research into the development of healthy parent and child relationships. There can also be unrecognised and unaddressed pre and perinatal (PPN) issues for both mum and child that can contribute to discord and disconnect. Although newborns and young babies may not be verbally equipped, their physical body does speak a formative language, the signs and cues of their BBL, of wounds that are still there in the tissues and unconscious domain which we understand can be a feeding ground for the roots of emotional disconnect.

A common circumstance, and one that can be more readily recognisable, is during the delivery when the birthing baby and mum may have lost some degree of emotional connection with each other. For example, a young child may appear very frustrated and angry towards his mum and strike out at her. This behaviour may have been played out since his babyhood as his perception (or resulting early imprint) was that mum "deserted me" by appearing not to be fully present for him during an intense and challenging part of his delivery.

Equally, mum might be harbouring feelings of undeclared guilt and regret around her child's delivery. Perhaps there was a medical intervention, such as an epidural administered for pain relief and an emergency assisted delivery as in the use of forceps or a caesarean section. Often these types of deliveries were not planned nor expected, resulting in a mum having to withdraw emotionally whilst she dealt with the overwhelm of the situation, then relief from the enduring labour pains and safe delivery of the baby. The feelings of guilt may also have been associated with the realisation around the possible negative impact her newborn could have experienced during the delivery, given the signs of his distress at birth, such as in his painful first cry, his distressed facial expression, the blue hue of his skin colour and evidence of facial bruising. These opposing perceptions of a baby/child and mum around the birthing experience can become more polarised with time as adaptive behaviours develop which then can become more ingrained as the child gets older and the dyad[6] relationship skews out of sync.

---

*Have you ever felt the desire for the world just to stop*
*for a little while?*
***Anne Matthews***

---

A helpful analogy for the parents and child is to offer an opportunity to stop and get off the emotionally laden merry-go-round of life; to take a time-out, to pause, reflect and regroup. This pacing of parents can be in the form of a facilitated conversation, with each parent sharing their perceived experiences of the pregnancy, labour, birth and of their newborn, together with presenting them with an interpretation of the child's BBL relating to his experience of the same. Encouraging and pacing parents to pause and review what happened and where the emotional disconnect may have occurred during the pregnancy, birth and in early days of their newborn, can be transformational in their family life. For example, consider this scenario; a mum may recall the specific moment when she felt she could no longer manage the pains of labour coupled with her distress for the safety of her baby who got stuck, stalling the delivery, all of which scared her. The baby would have been aware of his mum's distress coupled with how he experienced his own unique birthing journey in which he was unable to move forward, wary of the feelings of being compressed and stuck. Meanwhile, dad may have felt adrift as he

---

[6] Two individuals sustaining a sociologically significant relationship e.g. a parent and child

was unable to contribute meaningfully at the delivery, as the medical staff were more focused on his pregnant wife. Both labour and delivery can be a rollercoaster of emotions with parents tending not to revisit that time as the newborn and mum become the immediate focus of attention. As a result, the combination of anguish of a mum, dad and baby can be suppressed in the family's melting pot of past emotions.

Unaddressed issues from labour and birth from either the baby's or mum's perspective can become a narrative that then develops into a belief system. These early narratives are used to explain a baby's behaviour and parenting style. For example, the baby was always a bad sleeper; breastfeeding never worked for me. Such unaddressed issues tend to be repeated in subsequent pregnancies and deliveries. They can also be a reason for a mum not wanting to become pregnant again.

Facilitated sharing of the pregnancy and birth story by listening and understanding in an empathetic way enables a child, mum, and dad to get back in sync as they regroup and work from the same page of respecting and understanding the sequence of events that delivered their baby safely. This facilitated process of pacing helps gel the growing relationship of honouring the fear, distress, guilt and trauma and replacing it with a healing and evolving relationship as they move forward together as a united front. It enables everyone to have a sense of compassion and empathy around what they may have experienced without any judgement. This then proceeds with a realistic understanding upon which a trusting relationship can be celebrated between the baby/child, mum and dad. Otherwise, in my experience, relationships can become contaminated by misplaced fear, guilt and regret which can be detrimental to the building blocks of bonding and attachment of baby and mum, and with dad.

Beliefs that a newborn can be spoilt by being held and cuddled too much; that the baby will only settle for mum and not dad; that co-sleeping is bad for babies; that babies don't need to be breastfed; that babies shouldn't cry; that babies should not be wakeful; that white noise is good for babies, etc. are often perpetuated when the negative aspects surrounding a child's PPN experiences and those of parents are left unheard and unaddressed.

Furthermore, an interruption to the baby's normal sequence of development from their reflexive movements in the womb and during delivery has the potential to delay a baby's development in their early years. These children can be identified as not meeting their milestones as seen in the children described as skipping their four-point crawling stage and doing commando-style crawling instead; or the children that parents describe as slow to walk, slow to talk and difficult to potty train, to name a few. In these cases, the unique settings of the child's NS, which determines a child's natural pacing in life, can be out of kilter. This is something that a child is often very aware of and will seek to let a parent know from the beginning as a newborn and will continue until they are heard! We commonly see this to be the case in wakeful and unsettled babies, those with digestive and bowel issues, children with anxiety issues and those who are described as being needy, demanding or controlling.

## The Elephant in the Room

The situations cited above may resonate with you as it is only when we, as parents, are challenged in this way that we truly realise that we were blind to the emotional disconnection that exists between us and our baby, perhaps from which few of us escape! In my clinical experience, this can often be the elephant in the room that needs to be named and understood in the early treatment sessions of building trust and rapport. Pacing and choosing the optimal moment to bring this particular nugget to mum's and dad's attention is often a welcome relief, both to them and to the baby or child too. Grasping this concept is about guiding and pacing parents in honing their skills to understand and interpret their child's BBL, from their repetitive behaviour patterns *and* how we, as a mum or dad, are emotionally triggered and may tend to overreact rather than respond from an informed and grounded place of awareness. Being honest and very gentle with yourself on this journey of self-discovery and transformation with your child can be life-changing.

In my clinical experience, any signs of a child's early resistance to therapy in a session usually highlight that the parents may, on some level, be approaching the session from the perspective that the child needs fixing in some way. If this is the case, I then need to loop back and connect with mum, for example, and pace her needs. Usually, something has shifted and a new undeclared emotion may have arisen which the child has detected and is letting me know.

### What is the default setting of your child's nervous system?

Let us take a small detour to learn a little about the basic functions of our nervous system and how it expresses and integrates the body's sensory and motor systems. This prepares the landscape for parents to read and interpret their child's BBL, so please stay with me for this valuable next piece. It is important to realise that the brain and NS play a role in every aspect of our health and wellbeing. Together, they guide everyday activities such as waking up, walking and running; automatic activities such as our heart pumping blood around the body, breathing and digesting and more complex processes such as thinking, reading, remembering and feeling emotions.

The involuntary (or autonomic) part of the NS automatically interprets the information coming in from our senses (our sensory system) which it then expresses in terms of how we display our everyday feelings, emotions and behaviour. In fact, this is reflected in how we tell our story about who we are, what we think and how we view the world around us. The brain takes this information and creates a narrative, our story, to make sense of what is happening in the body.

The working mode of a child's nervous system is operating very early in the baby's development in the womb and then reset at birth. It will tend to default to those settings, especially at times when he feels distressed.

The tricky bit for parents is reading their baby's BBL and getting what they are telling us! The following steps can help us to understand the process:

- interpreting and understanding the story that our baby or child is telling involves us reading the "present emotional or physiological state" of their BBL e.g. noticing their feelings of overwhelm, loneliness or despair;

- facilitating an emotional or physiological "state change" for the baby/child by responding to their needs in the moment; and

- recognising and acknowledging any updated state of their BBL e.g. feeling safe or socially engaged.

Please take a few minutes to study the State Change diagram (next page) on the hourglass effect which helps to illustrate the neurophysiology of how a child's behavioural state can transition - through state changes. For example, from the 'present state' of feeling restrictive and limiting, through the window of tolerance in which change can be facilitated, to become expansive and curious.

In doing so a child can move from the shock, fear and a shutdown phase, to an emotional state where he can feel safe, socially engaged and connected. When this transition to an empowered state, the brain and NS are rewired from the 'old' pattern of overwhelm and despair. A child's NS will move to an updated state of "I can do ".

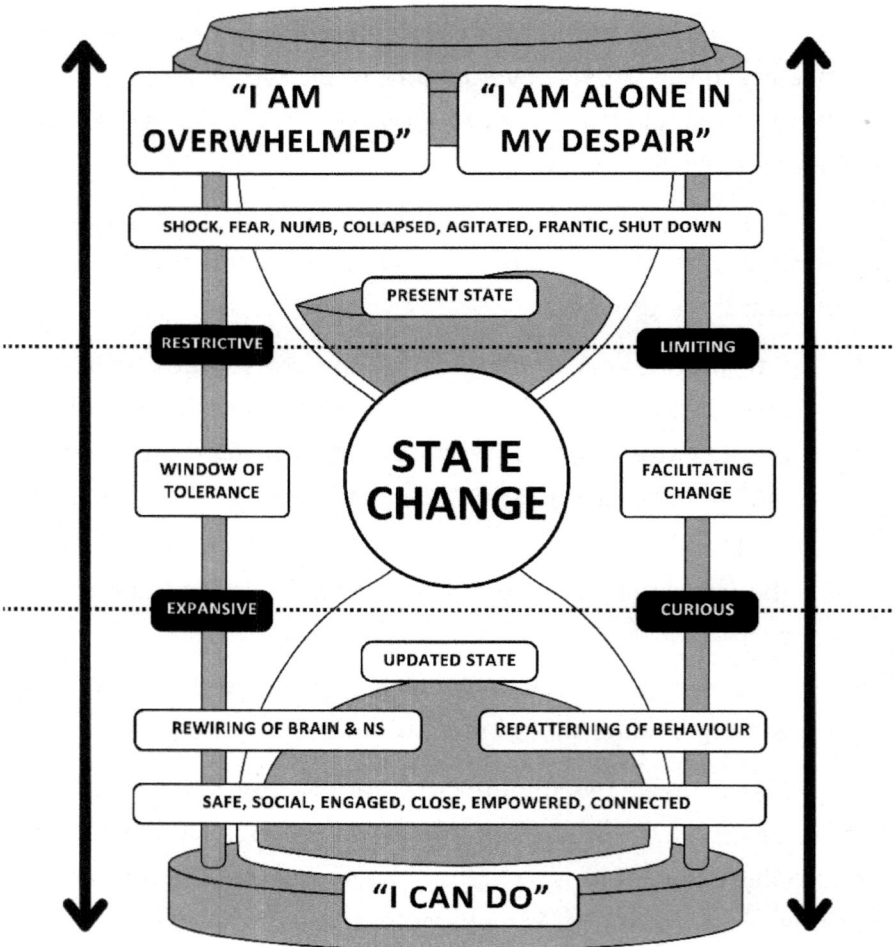

An hourglass diagram illustrating state change. Top section: "I AM OVERWHELMED" and "I AM ALONE IN MY DESPAIR". Below: SHOCK, FEAR, NUMB, COLLAPSED, AGITATED, FRANTIC, SHUT DOWN. PRESENT STATE. Left: RESTRICTIVE; Right: LIMITING. Middle: WINDOW OF TOLERANCE, STATE CHANGE, FACILITATING CHANGE. Left: EXPANSIVE; Right: CURIOUS. UPDATED STATE. REWIRING OF BRAIN & NS, REPATTERNING OF BEHAVIOUR. SAFE, SOCIAL, ENGAGED, CLOSE, EMPOWERED, CONNECTED. Bottom: "I CAN DO".

The facilitation of a state change effectively rewires the child's brain and NS allowing them to operate more efficiently and productively, as they integrate the new information, reducing the child's old defensive and adaptive behaviours. There are several steps in the process of facilitating a state change, many of which will unfold in the next few pages as you read the stories of parents of children with challenging or defensive type behaviours.

### Tommy, aged three years

### The Parents' Story

*"Tommy was born when our family lived in New Zealand, which is where his dad, Isaac, was born. We decided to return to my hometown in Northern Ireland when Tommy was two years old after he had been diagnosed with permanent hearing loss. When he was three years old, we were referred to Anne because we had been told that Tommy's problems were chronic and he needed to be supported with sensory integration. We were unsure what that meant but we trusted the therapist who referred us and we made the initial appointment.*

*"Before we met with Anne, we had a 15-minute appointment with a National Health Service speech and language therapist who made a diagnosis of autism and said that Tommy would be severely impaired. As his mum, and as someone who works within the health service, I understood the pressure of such a short appointment, and I was concerned that I had not been able to properly advocate for Tommy but was most concerned that this diagnosis did not feel correct for my son. We decided to learn as much as we could just in case it was correct but the stories we heard and the parents that we met seemed to be having many different experiences to us. We also believed that Tommy's profound and permanent hearing loss needed to be further considered and adjusted for.*

"Isaac had not been able to stay in Northern Ireland with us as he was still waiting for a visa and the necessary paperwork to be able to join us permanently so was not able to attend the initial appointment with Anne, but I called him immediately afterwards, filled with relief and renewed hope. Why? I knew that something was going to happen. Anne gave me hope that, together, we could unravel what Tommy was experiencing and, in a sense, build him again from the ground up. Anne helped us to change the vision for Tommy and, as opposed to special schools and limiting our expectations, we were now focused on Tommy's baby body language and development milestones. After that first appointment, he started to sleep and is now a child who has become at peace most of the time.

"If we can show you Tommy's trajectory over the next few years; when we first started on this journey with him, he was a small toddler of two years and one of the first therapists we went to who correctly identified that he appeared as a child trapped in a permanent state of unrest. When we first met Anne, he was at a point where, if he went into a room, he would wreck the room. He was like a whirlwind. We learned that he had not had time to develop because he was in a permanent state of panic, stuck in the limbo of fight or flight. The first thing that Anne taught me, as his mum, was to massage his neck and look into his eyes to connect with him.

"Tommy and Anne quickly developed a relationship of respect. When he knew he was going to visit Anne, he visibly relaxed. There is such a sense of calm within the treatment room and that sense of calm carries on after the appointments which we saw in his increasing capacity to sit still for longer periods of time. At nursery school, he was then able to sit still for up to ninety minutes.

"As parents, we learned about the benefits of physical alignment, and the importance of vagal tone, for a child's development and ability to be happy, relaxed and content.

"In the pre-Anne days, he didn't want to sit or stand on sand or grass and seemed to find it impossible to be still. After two years, he was more relaxed and able to sit still, he could count his numbers and tell the time. It is such a relief – we always knew he had that potential. In learning about his baby body language, exercise and nutrition, we have been able to support Tommy so that he has repeated nursery school and is now going into primary school with a classroom assistant.

"Our vision now is focused on building Tommy's speech and ability to communicate with the other kids in his class - he loves to play with other children and we see him trying to fit in. He is always wanting outside to play now and plays well with other children who invite him along to their birthday parties. It is in his speech that we have seen great progress as he has hundreds of words and we are helping him to use them to construct sentences.

"For him to be able to develop his fine motor skills, we had to first support him to develop fully those gross motor skills through physical activity by walking, climbing, jumping and balancing on his bicycle. One of the best buys was a trampoline; his auditory specialist told us that all hearing aids should come with a trampoline!

"We must confess that, due to all the problems and issues Tommy was facing, he was being let away with everything or "blue murder," as we would term it. Anne not only helped us to know what help Tommy needed, she gave us the gift of boundaries. As boundaries were enforced, and sometimes they still needed to be revisited, Tommy got more comfortable. The boundaries helped us all to contain behaviours and, although we may regress at times, this remains an area of focus. Boundaries have allowed us to gain trust and calm again within the home. They have been very powerful in enabling a better relationship between Tommy and his older sister, Sarah. Their relationship has become warm and they now really engage when they play together. Previously, she was at times neglected as we followed Tommy around the house putting out proverbial fires and we would find her alone reading. Now the books have become a shared joy and she will read to Tommy who now wants to read her books.

"Our family life is calmer, Tommy is an active child, he has good relationships with his sibling and peers, and he wants to learn! He is learning and we are learning together as a family."

## Recognising BBL

Julia and Isaac are loving and committed parents who were keen to understand and manage the impact of their son Tommy's early emotional imprints, his diagnosis of profound hearing loss and global developmental delay, together with the help of his older sister, Sarah. Firstly, they learned to recognise aspects of his BBL such as the hyper-defensive pattern that their son's imbalanced brain and NS were calibrated at. Secondly, they recognised the importance of providing a safe environment for Tommy where he could grow and develop as he discovered the joys of playing outdoors. Effectively, they were facilitating a "state change" from his "old" patterns. Thirdly, they tracked his BBL state changes by practising the element of looping back and reviewing his changing needs in the present. This, together with setting boundaries, helped him to develop secure emotional attachments and wholesome connections with his parents, and other carers, as he caught up on his developmental milestones.

At the family's first session, three-year-old Tommy looked like he was "out of it" as he struggled to stand still, wobbling back and forth on his thin legs and hyperextended knees that bent backwards.

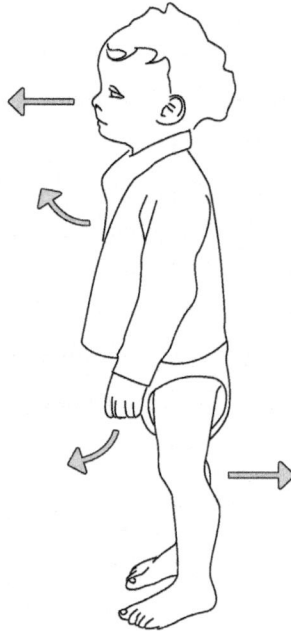

Tommy looked dazed and had difficulty keeping his slumped head and neck upright on his shoulders. He scanned me and the treatment room as if trying to make sense of where he was. Although Tommy was non-verbal, he screamed a lot in a high-pitched tone. It was readily obvious from his posture that he had weak core muscle tone and his incredibly pale pallor was as white as the milk in his bottle, which he sucked to self-soothe, as he settled on his mum's lap.

Tommy's lack of hearing was noticed shortly after birth but his hearing loss would not be formally diagnosed until he was two years old. His mum, Julia, readily became both his advocate and his protector over the next three years. Hearing loss meant that, although Tommy missed out on many aspects of normal development in the womb, his developing nervous system adapted and compensated by developing extra sensory awareness in other areas. Tommy appeared to have developed a sharp sense around touch, vibration and sight which mum was very aware of. As a result, Julia appeared to know Tommy's every move and knew when he needed to be hugged and cuddled after an outburst and when he wanted to be left alone. However, his range of adaptive behaviours was becoming increasingly difficult to manage at home as Tommy needed constant attention and supervision during his wakeful hours in order not to harm himself or others. Mum was also cognisant of Tommy's neurodevelopmental delay as he was not meeting his developmental milestones around feeding, dressing, interacting and playing.

### Pacing a hyper-sensitive child

As Tommy was an acutely sensitive child, pacing his sensory needs was critical to allow him to express and download his emotions. He seemed to initiate his own healing process during his therapy. In the early sessions, he would weep deeply, unprompted, and either flop or flail his limbs in anguish as mum shared significant parts of his life story. This gave him an opportunity to release some of the emotional patterns from his experiences in the womb and at birth.

The somato emotional release that he made through his gestures and crying would start as soon as he entered the treatment room. Tommy sensed that I understood his Baby Body Language and that mum was his advocate. Secondly, he recognised that his Baby Body Language was being understood, read, interpreted and managed positively for him. It was like "he cut to the chase" and got on with downloading his emotions after which he would feel better and mum would record his progress in daily activities at home. Keeping a progress journal to record a child's progress is important for parents. They can refer back to it, especially at times when they feel that they've reached a plateau.

Tommy allowed his parents to share specific aspects of his life story. I would gently call a pause and pace mum's sharing of her story at the earliest signs of intense emotional moments for either one of them. This facilitation process helped to interpret and explain how Tommy and mum might have experienced things in the past by tuning into how the story was resonating with them in the present moment.

These experiences (or early imprints) would shed light on what Tommy may have experienced in the womb; in that warm and softly coloured womb where he was being caressed, held and supported as he moved around with ease, sensing the comforting vibrations from his mum's voice, internal plumbing and bodily movements and the voices and energies of others around her. Imagine the shocking transition from the solitude of a trusting womb into a busy, intense delivery room with bright lights and well-meaning medical staff handling the baby in an efficient and hurried way.

Imagine how the highly charged emotions of fear and worry from his mum and dad during the difficult labour and birth were lodged into his nervous system at this critical stage in his development. The intense attention and urgency from the obstetric team would also have had their impact and lodged in Tommy's fragile nervous system. How he also imprinted the highly charged, stressful fears and emotions his mum and dad reported during the labour, and the intense attention from the obstetric team, would have been registered in his early imprint narrative.

## "My baby held up his head from day one"

Mum described how she had felt an overwhelming sense of panic when the midwives suspected that the umbilical cord was around Tommy's neck at the final stages of labour. His head was not moving through the cervix. He was stuck. Tommy would have felt his mum's sense of panic, together with what he was experiencing physically and emotionally from the strangulation pressure on his neck, and his head being compressed and stuck in the birth canal.

On delivery, Julia reported how Tommy had "held up his head from day one", a description which is of great concern for me as this equates to a baby that may have experienced significant physical and emotional birth trauma. Tommy's NS had gone into a fight/flight reaction, characterised by his reported state of hyper-alertness with taut overactive neck muscles and upright head posture, which is not in keeping with the expected developmental stage of a newborn baby.

From a BBL perspective, this is usually an indicator that the baby's head, neck and shoulders were physically compromised due to the mechanical effects of compression of the head on the neck and shoulders, with restriction around the neck, throat and airways. Julia met her newborn son with a look of panic etched on his face. This facial expression of panic and distress quickly turned to inconsolable crying. Some babies can be so deeply shocked that they are silent at birth. In such cases, the baby's breathing rhythm is usually also affected as it tends to be rapid and shallow. Parents will often report that their baby had a history of recurrent chest infections in early babyhood. This could be because the baby would have been struggling to take adequate and deep enough breaths to clear the secretions from their lungs.

Incidentally, this apparent "strong neck" in newborns has been reported in many babies delivered during the Covid-19 pandemic when mums-to-be were under tremendous pressure and stress during their pregnancy, delivery and at birth for a variety of reasons.

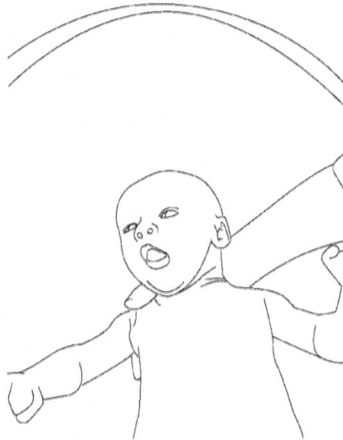

Stress hormones, such as cortisol, would have been consistently high under such circumstances which directly affects the developing brain of the foetus. This causes natural and intelligent adaptations by the baby whose NS has had to adapt to survive e.g. an in-built fear around sleeping and settling.

### The impact of head and jaw misalignment

The way the head is positioned on the neck is controlled by the neck muscles which are attached to the upper chest and shoulders. Positioning of the head dictates how symmetrically the muscles of the jaw joint work; the skull needs to rock back and forth, ever so slightly, for the jaw joints to work synchronously. The jaw joints are unique in that they are the only joints in the body that are designed to always move simultaneously in three different directions. Firstly, they can move the jaw up and down by opening and closing the mouth. Secondly, they can glide the lower jaw forwards and backwards and, thirdly, side to side. These movements develop very early on in life to allow swallowing, sucking and then chewing and will become more efficient as the child develops. The scaffolding effect of the neck, shoulder muscles and spine must support the head adequately for these jaw joints to work efficiently. In Tommy's case, his head was tilted forward with his neck muscles taut and tight. This can be scary for a child because it feels to them like they are constantly on the point of tipping over. A child in this state would be constantly on alert and unable to relax, with little interest in eating or feeding himself due to his distracted state of being.

One of the first things that needed to be addressed was the mobility and strength of Tommy's spine, pelvic and shoulder areas so that he could start to support his head more efficiently on his shoulders. When a child is feeling more coordinated, balanced and has greater stamina, his interest in food will often improve because he is feeling more comfortable. Understandably, Tommy also had great difficulty settling for sleep during the day or night due to his NS being stuck in a high alert mode. As he had been unable to release the tension around his neck and shoulders, his adapted behaviour was one of continuous movement that had become very familiar to his parents.

Tommy's medical paediatric team and other professionals had diagnosed him with global neurodevelopmental delay, heightened Moro[7] Reflex and asthma, requiring the use of an inhaler for an ongoing viral wheeze.

---

[7] The Moro Reflex is an infantile reflex that develops between 28-32 weeks gestation and normally disappears at 3-6 months of age. It is the visible as baby will spread their arms out then pull their arms back in and cry.

Although this was an accurate medical reflection of Tommy's symptoms, my work was helping his parents find the answers to why his NS had responded in that way. His survival strategy was to keep moving in a bid to move away from his pain, discomfort and fear due to his NS being on high alert but, for a three-year-old whose natural blueprint is to meet his developmental milestones, this situation was like having one foot on the brake and the other on the accelerator at the same time. He was trying to move forward developmentally and he was screeching to a stop at the same time! He was continuously frustrated.

Tommy was referred to me by a local neuro-developmental therapist who was helping him to progress from his retained Moro Reflex. We each refer clients to one another, as we repeatedly see evidence of the benefits of each other's work in the progress of the children who attend us.

From my expertise and experience of working with children with neurodevelopmental dysfunction, my intention was to reset his NS by, firstly, taking the physical pressure off Tommy's head, neck and shoulders. Musculoskeletal pressure and restriction were depleting the resilience of both his nervous and immune systems and were preventing him from progressing in other areas of co-development.

### Getting on the same page

Tommy's adaptive behaviours were causing constant anxiety and interrupting his developmental progress, particularly around speech, language, and social engagement. Tommy's interest in food and feeding himself were also very limited as his high alert NS was craving quick carbs which would give him instant energy. His nutrition was limited to milk, pasta, bread and cereal which is typical for children like him. Furthermore, because of Tommy's cranial compression issues, sucking a bottle while lying on his back, with his head and neck extended over his mum's lap, was facilitating a gentle rhythmic movement of his delicate spine and helping to ease the pressure on his cranial plates and developing brain. Observing Tommy's BBL patterns and having heard the collaborative story from his mum regarding his life in the womb, his delivery and birth story and the difficult time his parents had to settle him as a baby, the picture of how best to meet Tommy's needs became apparent.

The first step was to let Tommy know that he was being seen, heard and honoured with understanding and empathy for what he had experienced. As I coached Julia, she tuned into those feelings by hearing and sensing her son's plight in the present moment which increased her depth of awareness around Tommy's distress. This helped to shift them both towards greater connection and to heal his birth trauma. It is also the ideal place to begin to repair a disconnection between mum and baby. It involved leading and pacing Tommy, his mum and maternal grandma (who was also at the initial consultation) to a place of understanding and meaningful connection.

In a session, my focus is to relate to, pace, pause and settle the child and their parents. I review the progress that has been made by looping back every few steps as changes are made. Mirroring back a mum's narrative can help her shift awareness in understanding her child's behaviour as I pace her progress. Introducing a pause in a session by guiding a mum to check in with her breathing rhythm and to consciously follow her breath in and out is a valuable self-regulatory practice. This is a self-help technique that I coach parents in when they are feeling emotionally triggered when sharing their child's birth narrative or when the child expresses their dis-ease. This is the child's experience of their body not being at ease and when they resort to behaviours that are adaptive to their situation. Understandably, parents will perceive this as negative behaviour. So often, parents express difficulty finding strategies to manage their child's adaptive behaviours because they are unwittingly reacting against them, rather than understanding them from the BBL perspective.

### Adaptive behaviours

These strategies often arise out of some sort of fear or misunderstanding. A mum may feel fear or shame in anticipation of her child's misbehaviour and unpredictability at family gatherings or public settings. These feelings may be projected onto her child as they can sense their mum's triggered emotions. This triggers the child's adaptive behaviour to the situation and so a tit-for-tat cycle can emerge.

Guiding parents to engage with these unwanted feelings and emotions and to take ownership of them is part of the therapeutic process. It frees them to model emotional regulation and to be 'present in the moment' for their child. This enables a child to express their emotions and release their feelings from negative past experiences 'in the moment'. It is about interrupting the cycle of unwanted emotions and feelings and a parent is best able to settle her child by learning to co-regulate his NS in this way.

In early treatment sessions, some children are very triggered by the energetic and emotional field around the sharing of their birth narrative. They often react to their parents' emotional state by displaying their adaptive behaviour in a bid to discharge their tension patterns, such as being unable to stay still and wanting to touch, move and throw things in the room or strike out at a parent or sibling. Older children can be very verbal and express and direct their anger and frustrations towards a parent. My role is to meet a child and their parents where they need to be met as I pace and manage the intensity of their interactions and assess the primary problem.

## Home care and practical tips

Amusingly, in Tommy's case, he would soon let us know if we were off track or if he did not want something to be discussed in the room, particularly around my guidance in establishing more acceptable boundaries at home. Change can be challenging for both adults and children.

Coaching parents to set behavioural boundaries, in a compassionate and empathetic manner that paces the child as they develop their own sense of self-regulation and connectedness, is part of the therapeutic process. Resilience research indicates that ongoing interplay between the parents or caregiver and child promotes healthy brain development.

As the main focus at home was to help Tommy develop a greater connection between his physical body and his sensory system, I recommended mum to take him for a lengthy walk outdoors each day. I emphasised the need to introduce him to achievable challenges by starting with walking up gentle inclines and then progressing to climbing steep and rougher terrains.

The aim was to help Tommy experience what it was like to get out of breath, pause and recover. As his physical ability and stamina improved he repatterned his NS from being stuck in the fight/flight fear-driven mode. He was then able to take deeper breaths which helped him to regulate his NS. Fortunately, the family lived in a beautiful area of rugged glens and valleys. This outdoor activity allowed Tommy to feel more embodied by discovering the sensory delights of nature through the rugged landscape he viewed and the effect of the elements, the heat of the sun, the rain and wind against his skin. This naturally diverted some of the energy from his overloaded sensory system into his physical body and effectively discharged it into the ground.

Subsequently, this progress enabled essential shifts in other areas of his development including his verbal communication and how he related to the needs of other members of his family, including the cat who he had been terrorising by tail-pulling and kicking.

Dad had relocated from New Zealand by the time of Tommy's next session. Again, Tommy cried and became emotional as soon as he entered the treatment room. His parents reported that although their week had been filled with celebration parties Tommy had not coped well with the interruption to his daily routines. He readily allowed me to work around his head and shoulders and he calmed as he responded to my therapeutic touch. I encouraged his parents to consider their language when Tommy experienced intense emotions. I suggested the use of connecting language by using phrases like the following when responding to his adaptive and triggering behaviours.

**Connecting Language examples**
**"I see you."**
**"I am listening."**
**"I am here for you."**
**"I want to understand and sense what you are feeling."**

As the sessions progressed, Tommy showed that his NS felt safer, more regulated and more connected by curling up on the settee between his parents and continuing to absentmindedly self-soothe as he sucked at the teat of his bottle. It was very probable that Tommy had been aware of a level of anxiety and separation that his mum and sister had felt with dad being so far away. He too would have been processing and managing his emotions around the relief of the family being reunited in the early months of the Covid pandemic in Spring 2020.

Over the course of Tommy's treatment sessions, I guided Julia and Isaac to use practical tips and creative ideas at home. We started with basic massage techniques, which they continued to practise, and developed other self-help resources over a three-year period up to the time of writing this book.

When massaging, I guide parents to be mindful of their child's emotional threshold level by reading the physical signs of comfort; for example, gauging breathing rhythm, allowing a child to move around if they need to not expecting them to remain still whilst being massaged. Tommy's parents began recognising and connecting with their child's window of tolerance and facilitated a state change by forging trust and understanding, and strengthening the relationship with their child.

### Facilitating rebirthing

On building a trusting relationship with a family, a mum will normally share a story about a behaviour or habit that initially appears random to her but, in fact, these gems often have a great significance regarding both the child's interrupted developmental sequence and a parent's intuitiveness. Julia described the increasing frustration around mealtimes when Tommy would defiantly leave the table and seek out their winged wicker chair to play in, climb upside down and fiercely resist mum's attempts to bring him back to the kitchen table.

It became obvious to me, from his choice of play, that he needed to practise his rebirthing movements which were being misconstrued by mum as defiant behaviour and Tommy not wanting to sit at the table to eat at mealtime. Children often play out their rebirthing movements at a time when they have their mum's undivided attention which, of course, is usually not what a mum would necessarily have in mind at mealtimes!

I helped Julia practise this valuable rebirthing step with Tommy to reset the rhythm and integration of his interrupted developmental movement pattern. This involved supporting Tommy to hang vertically from his feet and ankles as he gradually relieved himself of tensions in his spine, neck and head. Julia repeated this with Tommy at home every day for the next four weeks.

This rebirthing inversion stretch is best performed by a parent over a cushioned surface of the floor or a sofa, depending on the age, height and weight of the child but not immediately after a meal.

To practise this manoeuvre with your child, use the following steps as guidance but, if you are not confident or need more explanation, please consult a BBL practitioner who will guide you further.

### Facilitating rebirthing movements with a child

### Inverted Hold

1.  Ask the child to lie down on their back as you make reassuring eye contact.

2.  Let them know that you are going to lift them up by their feet and ankles.

3.  Place your hands around the front of their ankles with your thumbs contacting their heels.

4.  Raise their legs only to a 90-degree right angle to their torso.

5.  Hold firmly to their ankles as you lift their legs upwards to raise their bottom off the floor.

6. Continue lifting smoothly until your child is hanging vertically with their head a few inches off the floor.

7. Pause and hold this position for 10-30 seconds while your child realigns and extends their head and stretches their arms outwards.

8. To come out of the position, lower their head slowly to gently touch the floor and move slowly backwards, as the child flexes their neck and head, and smoothly return them to the starting position.

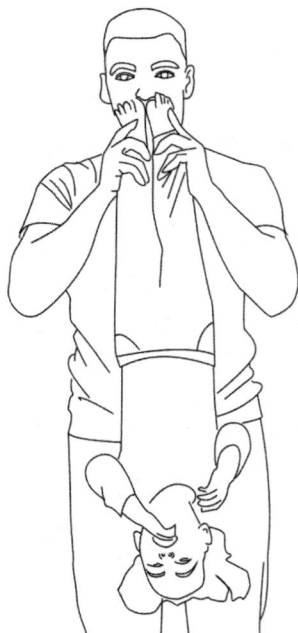

For the younger child, help them to focus by counting aloud slowly from one to three as you raise them up through positions 4, 5 and 6.

Be confident and reassuring as you hold and support your child through steps 1 to 5 until your child is ready to move into the full vertical hold position.

Repeat the full inverted hold three times and notice how your child's NS processes and releases with each hold. Continue this daily practice until your child moves effortlessly into the vertical position, extends their head and neck, relaxes their arms and enjoys the full stretch. Children will often prompt you when they sense that they need this inverted spinal stretch - so look out for that!

### Facilitating rebirthing movements with a baby

1. For babies, it is preferable to lie them across a Swiss ball, on their tummy.

2. Keep a firm hold on the waistband of their clothing whilst rolling the ball slowly back and forth and then side to side. This action will activate the extensor muscles of their back and neck and help them extend in a similar way to the inverted stretch.

3. Repeat daily and monitor progress until your baby is able to easily open into a full body stretch with head and neck extended and arms outstretched.

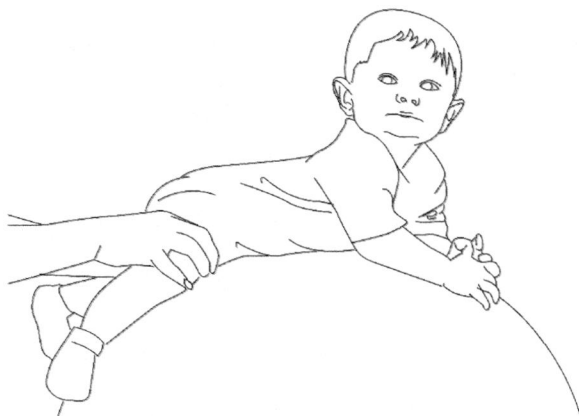

Children whose NS and spinal alignment are out of balance will initially have a defensive reluctance to the stretch. With gradual progression of the manoeuvre, the child will release the spinal tension and breathe more deeply and efficiently as their brain and NS integrate the changes.

This inverted hold exercise has a powerful calming effect on the NS and calms sensory-related meltdowns that children can have.

Some children will appear skewed as the asymmetry in their spine becomes obvious in the inverted position. With practice, this will lessen although the child may require some manual bodywork correction from a professional if the asymmetry persists.

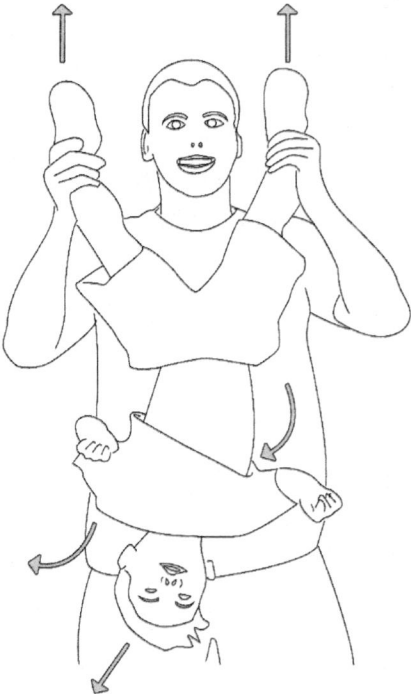

Children will also seek this rebalancing activity out in the play park by hanging upside down from the play equipment by themselves.

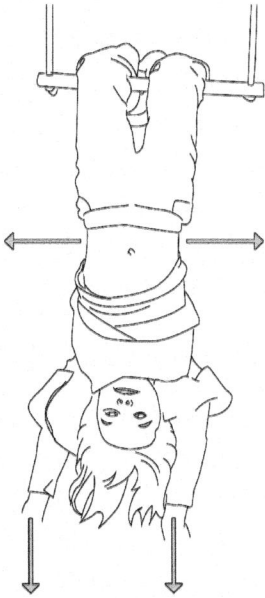

They will also lie over a Swiss ball or over the side of a bed or couch, as it makes them feel good.

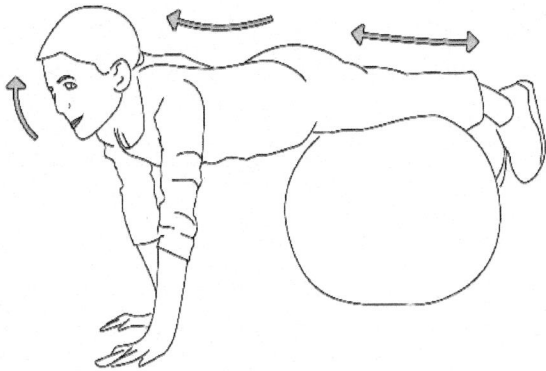

## Hanging Out Upside Down

In Tommy's case, his parents immediately noted that the inverted hold exercise calmed his NS and lessened the frequency of the sensory-related meltdowns that he was having, due to being overwhelmed. Julia was encouraged to keep light physical contact with Tommy's back or tummy, as he lay on the floor after these stretches, giving him the necessary time to process the *state change* that he was experiencing as he re-patterned the rebirthing movement into his brain and NS. This was another step in his developmental progress and offered expansion and release throughout his body.

## The perinatal cues in babies

Breast or bottle-feeding mums will often mention how their hungry baby pulls off the breast or teat, for no apparent reason, just as they are about to feed. This can be explained in a similar way to Tommy's behaviour in the wicker chair. This situation tells us of a baby whose descent into the birth canal, and exit through the vagina, had been interrupted, for whatever good reason – in Tommy's case as a medical emergency due to the umbilical cord around his neck. The baby's blueprint for their own natural pacing and connection with mum's hormonally triggered contractions, during delivery and birth, would also have been interrupted. As a result, the baby will try to simulate that part of their innate journey again but in the manner and timing which they wanted and needed to do it. This can be tricky for mums who may misread their baby's BBL and jump to unhelpful conclusions such as the baby is rejecting mum, is not hungry or has wind, is no longer interested in breastfeeding or that mum is not maternal enough. In my practice, I hear these reasons and many more from mums and dads!

The most common mum and baby-related frustrations and angst are around feeding and digestion issues. When the baby was in the womb, he was feeding on demand directly from the umbilical cord together with having his mum's constant attention and connection. Understandably, babies and young children might have an expectation that it will be the same on the outside! Unfortunately, mums are not always guided to be mindful of this reality from the baby's perspective and, therefore, the concept of viewing the first year of life as being the fourth trimester is very useful. Supporting a mum in this way eases the transition for mum and baby and gives a greater regard to the impact of the early imprints that the newborn has experienced.

There is a strong association between the issues of feeding, bonding and attachment between mum and baby and the baby or child's instinct to reset the NS from the effects of birth trauma. These are observable in reading and interpreting a baby or child's BBL.

In this situation, I invite a mum to facilitate the baby's movement, with positive intention, by placing one hand under the back of the baby's head and neck, allowing the baby to ease his head against her hand and gently follow the slow rhythmical turning and unwinding movements of his head, neck and upper body. She then gently places her other hand lightly over the upper part of his chest, creating a V-shape with her thumb and first finger and gently feeling an upward pressure from the baby as he extends and lengthens his upper body over the crook of her other arm.

The baby is effectively unwinding his fascial (internal connecting tissues) tension from the shock and restrictions that he has been holding in his body. One contributing factor is the compressional forces on the head and upper spine during birth, often at the most intense part of the vaginal delivery, and can be collaborated by mum's narrative of the birth story and how she felt during the labour. Commenting on her birth experiences, she will say phrases like, *"The labour was very long; the baby got stuck; the low back pain became too unbearable; I thought 'I can't do this', or I needed pain relief."*

This is usually the time when the baby's progress down the birth canal and through the cervix was interrupted. The baby may have felt fear or shock due to the intense compression of mum's pelvic bones on his head, face, neck and parts of his body. Although he is holding the emotional tension of this trauma in his body, he instinctively needs to expand, heal and move forward with his development. The restrictions tend to hold a baby back from feeding comfortably and digesting efficiently. There is no better person than his mum to re-enact this drama with, given that his perception would be that she was part of his early experience. There is no blame or shame; that is just the way it was.

Babies are very forgiving and resilient; they want to move on and offload their delivery, birthing tension and restriction patterns. They only become confused or frustrated when mum appears to ignore their BBL cues of wanting to release these early imprints and seems to only focus on their symptoms of wind, colic, constipation, wakefulness, etc. Taking the problem-solving approach, and searching for the cause of their discomfort by listening to their birth narrative, is the key for bonding and attachment that mum and baby address by reconnecting on their healing journey.

### A Parents' Guide

I continued to top up the contents of Julia and Isaac's backpack of guidance tips and tools over the course of Tommy's progress, which they keenly and enthusiastically accepted. Julia continued to facilitate Tommy's cues for practising his rebirthing stretches to regulate his NS and his desire to play outdoors and partake in a range of physical activities. I also instructed and demonstrated how to progress the technique of gently but firmly massaging across his shoulder muscles and at the prominent slender muscles at the side of his neck together with brushing his hair as if massaging his head along and around his cranial suture lines. Hypersensitive children prefer a strong contact rather than a light touch massage as otherwise, it feels tickly and unpleasant.

## Progressing to Social Engagement Mode

For children like Tommy, it is imperative to facilitate a shift of their NS out of a fixed fight/flight mode to allow access to the social engagement part of the NS. This aids brain recovery and assists with their coordination and balance development by improving the ability to connect with their core, midline and the symmetrical movement of all four limbs. As more parts of the brain are accessed, which were previously closed, it opens the creative and learning gates for children. As Tommy's adaptive fear pattern settled, he quickly showed signs of being a very intelligent child who was readily able to recognise and create three-digit numbers when asked. In fact, he loved the challenge of doing them. However, the sensory and emotional parts of his brain also needed to catch up with this intellectual development which would be part of his future neurodevelopmental exercise programme.

Julia and Isaac began to observe that Tommy was bottle feeding more at times when he needed to settle and self-soothe after an outburst of frustration or when they anticipated that they needed to avoid an emotional meltdown and sensed that he was fear-driven. This situation also coincided with Tommy becoming interested in foods that required more chewing and his parents were able to move away from offering him soft "nursery" type foods. Oral development and sensory issues around his connection with his fingers, hands and his mouth were improving and the bottle feeding finally came to an end around five years of age. As Tommy's nervous system was less on alert and his brain-to-gut feedback pathways were developing, he became more interested in meals and shared family meal times became an enjoyable social gathering.

Over the next few sessions, we learned that Tommy loved spinning in a chair, bouncing on the trampoline, sought out horseplay with his dad, loved being tumbled and held upside down by his feet and became much more interested in seeking out playtime with his sister who was interacting with him more too. Their sibling relationship had been affected by Tommy's developmental delays. However, his sister Sarah's relationships across the whole family had also been deeply affected. As is all too often the case, Sarah had learned to cope with her young brother's needs, and her parents' distraction, by increasingly seeking less and less attention to the point that she had come to be most often found reading and removing herself from the family to spend time alone. Her room and space were often invaded by Tommy and her needs had been neglected.

Sarah quickly responded to the positive changes within the family and, as his behaviour started to change, she found a new role with Tommy, as outlined above, by sharing her books and reading to him. There would also be increasing space and attention for Sarah with her father's return and her mum now having some more time and availability for her daughter. This is often part of a family's journey and, as things resolve, each member of the family, including siblings, has greater opportunity to have their needs met and find increasing levels of connection. All suggested that Tommy was moving away from his fearful fight/flight mode and was learning and seeking out ways in which to regulate his nervous system as different parts of his brain developed further. These were very positive signs of self-regulation which his parents honoured and welcomed with gratitude. I encourage parents to pause, reflect and loop back on their child's progress, to recognise and truly appreciate the marvellous capability of the plasticity, growth and recovery of the brain. A child's brain continues to develop to the age of 25 years so it is never too late to help your child.

As with all children, it is important to also consider the bigger picture and any other implications that might be happening in a child's life. For example, Tommy at one point began choosing to wear his left hearing aid only. We, therefore, questioned if the right was set at an incorrect pitch for him. I am keen to review things holistically, problem-solve and integrate other activities or disciplines parents might use to help a child's overall wellbeing.

This problem-solving approach supports parents because sometimes they can have doubts as to whether they should question another professional's opinion or ask them to review their child's situation. Also, there are a range of practical and logistical considerations to prepare when attending a medical appointment. For Tommy, it was also very challenging for him to have his ears touched. Mum and dad really benefitted from giving themselves permission to query when to attend, or even request, follow-up appointments rather than it just being a routine exercise. This is important when working with children as their needs can fluctuate and change very rapidly.

In this instance, where there was an obvious and new disparity in Tommy's comfort levels in the two hearing aids, Julia and Isaac were much more confident about requesting a review with the audiologist even though they had one recently.

Tommy was due to start nursery school and it was necessary to facilitate an interest around self-care activities such as dressing and undressing, washing hands and brushing teeth. As progress and change pave the way, the next step was creating distinct boundaries at home around acceptable and caring behaviour. Julia and Isaac agreed on the most challenging behaviours to focus on which we decided to review specifically at monthly appointments. For example, Tommy would react badly to the word "no" when he was doing something that his parents didn't want him to do. These situations triggered negative behaviour such as screaming and striking out, usually at mum. Julia understandably found this behaviour very difficult to handle and emotionally distressing, especially in public. On discussing these situations, I learned that Julia was also supporting two adult family members at home who had ongoing health issues.

Both parents acknowledged that with the added family distractions Tommy was allowed to get away with misbehaving as, often, it was a matter of taking the path of least resistance. In situations like this, I encourage parents to choose no more than three behavioural issues which are causing greatest havoc within the family dynamic. Both parents and the immediate carers need to agree on committing to a plan of action and maintaining it. However, parents need to play their part too because change comes from not just one person but from the dynamic between them. There also needs to be a "give and take" approach which Tommy had not yet developed.

I coached Julia on becoming more aware of how and when she was being triggered by Tommy's outbursts. She confessed to ongoing feelings of fear and shame and that she worried a lot about his future. Julia practised being less emotionally attached to Tommy's behaviour at the time of his outbursts by becoming more grounded and present in that moment. I demonstrated to Julia how to work on her own body language as I suspected that Tommy was receiving mixed messages from her which he was unable to understand and process at this stage. I advised mum to act out the message that she wanted to convey to Tommy by practising standing balanced and upright opposite Tommy, ready to raise her hands and arms to gesticulate and sign language "no" assertively by moving her hands sharply out in front of her chest. Holding her arms there as she repeated a firm "no", whilst maintaining a steady neutral gaze, would help to pace Tommy until he registered her intention.

When a child's NS is in flight mode, they are very internally focused and unable to immediately relate to another person's perspective. Doing something that the child would not expect you to do will stimulate their sense of curiosity and redirect their focus. This is one of the discovery keys that will shift the child's NS from their own internal world and switch tracks to stimulate the calm-inducing part of the NS and prepare the path to social engagement. Using the hook of curiosity prepares the child to pause in the moment, activates their awareness and helps them to shift gears from their fight/flight response and regulate their NS to become calmer and more socially engaged. The child moves from being stuck revving in second gear to shifting through the gears and cruising along in fifth into social engagement mode; a more efficient and more receptive place for the NS to travel in.

When a child progresses through the normal developmental sequence, from the womb and as a newborn, the apparent random movement of their body, limbs and head gives feedback to the brain as to how they are feeling and perceiving those around them. This feedback helps the various parts of the brain to expand, develop and connect at different times as they integrate and work with each other. When this sequence is interrupted, the blueprint for the developing brain is skewed.

In Tommy's case, his fight/flight response was firing repetitively with very little being learned from his experiences in terms of maturing in an age-appropriate way. His parents were also reacting to his fixed fear-driven fight/flight setting which was becoming increasingly reinforced as he got older. We needed to employ this circuit breaker approach to help Tommy's NS get back onto his developmental sequence to allow him to flourish. In doing so, he would receive a clear, strong message that his mum wanted him to listen to her and that hitting mum was not acceptable behaviour. This approach took a few days of practice as mum became more confident and Tommy responded with fewer outbursts as his NS found a new and more efficient way of working.

This approach was well-timed as Tommy was starting nursery school with one-to-one support and he adapted surprisingly well in interacting and following instructions from other adults whilst also being compliant about wearing his hearing aids. There was parallel progress at home as he developed an interest and capability in dressing himself. As a child develops in one area, we readily observe progress in other areas which is very encouraging to both parent and child. Tommy's physical stamina, balance and coordination improved and he was keen on learning to ride a bicycle with stabilisers which progressed to enjoying bonding cycle trips with his dad. Weekly swimming lessons on a one-to-one basis were also well received as he responded to the womb-like sensory and calming stimulation of floating.

These approaches gave Tommy a sense of safety, stoked his childlike curiosity and allowed him to become more self-aware and self-regulatory. Given his history of developmental delay, I supported his parents in their decision to successfully request their local educational authorities to allow Tommy to repeat another year at nursery school to help him catch up emotionally.

## Managing selective behaviour

As parents, we understand that children can behave differently with one parent compared to the other which can be difficult to manage and agree on. In Tommy's case, we had to review on how to manage his selective behaviour around seeking out his mum to hit when he experienced fear, anger or frustration, even when she was not in the same room as him. I suggested that Issac and Maria be more consistent in mirroring respect of personal physical boundaries consistently. Initially this involved Issac removing Tommy into another area of the house to discharge his feelings. As his NS became more regulated and less fear-driven, Tommy sought out a variety of physical outdoor play from bouncing on the trampoline to cycle rides with his dad.

As Tommy's biggest advocate, I recommended that Julia keep a journal to record his wins, progress and challenges and to regularly review it to remind herself and Isaac how much their son was progressing from the fear-driven state that he had been birthed into.

## Fear

When fear is triggered in our body, stress hormones are released into all our organs including our brain. Fear can displace our rational thoughts and is one of the most limiting emotions for children, as it interrupts their physical, emotional and intellectual development to varying degrees into adolescence and adulthood.

If you notice that you are becoming socially uncomfortable, especially in the presence of your child, and that you've mixed emotions ranging from anxiety, disappointment, anger, sadness, and frustration to regret, you may also be suffering from fear. For example, it might be a fear of what the future holds for your child and you, as a family.

The first step to every solution is acknowledgement and, when you notice fear bombarding your life, it's time to shift gears and make a change. As you dig deep and with self-compassion, place your main focus on what is truly valuable in your life. What are you grateful for? These are the early steps of releasing the fear that binds you. As you can focus more on living life, enjoying the moment and appreciating the abundance of opportunities that are right in front of you, your child and your family, fear will loosen its hold.

---

*"Everything you want is on the other side of fear."*
**Jack Canfield**

---

Consider that for a moment: to get what you want, you just need to get past your fear, as does your child.

I call upon you to become your own biggest supporter, not your own worst enemy. When you begin to acknowledge your capabilities, self-worth, self-esteem and confidence, others will notice - especially your children! Failure is inevitable in life and is a part of everyone's journey. It is up to you to take it in your stride, accept the lesson and let go of fear.

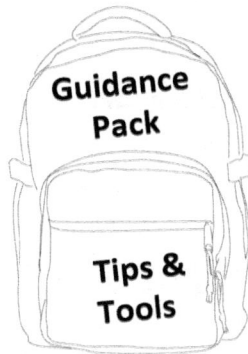

Guidance Pack

Tips & Tools

**"Lack of boundaries invites lack of respect."**

**Awareness**

**Six steps to help you pace your child and establish positive boundaries:**

- What are the signs of disconnect you notice in your child? For example, lacks eye contact, appears not to listen, is unable to stay still, has difficulty getting to sleep, is anxious, hits out at others.

- Continue with the basic nightly body massages as you help your child regulate their NS and build on the feelings of connection between you both. Tip: Use the opportunity to massage your child's head gently when shampooing their hair.

- As you feel more empowered, facilitate the rebirthing movements as described in this chapter. Tip: Allow your older child to hang out upside down on outdoor play equipment or over the sides of a sofa or Swiss ball.

- Regularly do something fun and light-hearted that your child would not be expecting. Surprise them as you trigger their curiosity which helps reset a shocked NS.

- Consider how you respond, rather than react, to your child and allow your response to act as a cycle breaker.

- As parents, agree on no more than two or three behaviours you want to address at any one time. Use your facial expressions, hand movements and body stance to reinforce your words as you give clear grounded instructions on your expectations. Be consistent and yet flexible as you facilitate positive change.

**Six steps to help recognise some of your own unaddressed issues:**

- Share your child's birth story with your partner or the significant other in their life.
- Practise taking turns to talk without being interrupted.
- Practise the art of active listening from your heart.
- Sense how you're feeling as you are seen and heard.
- Notice the words that you both repeatedly use in your narratives around your experiences of pregnancy, birth and first years of your child's life.
- How much fear, guilt, regret, despair, relief, resignation, happiness, and joy are you aware of?

## Reflections
**Consider these questions in your heart before answering:**

- How are you feeling just now?
- Where in your body do you feel those emotions?
- How do you think your child is feeling?
- When you sit for a few minutes with your emotions, how do you feel?
- How does it feel being seen and heard by your partner?
- Practise your 1:2 breathing as you record your thoughts in your journal.

# Chapter Three

## Building Trust and Rapport

The average age of children who first attend me is between three and six years of age. Parents will usually have sought help from elsewhere as they search for answers to address their child's challenges. They may have often lost hope and trust in their intuition, parenting skills and in finding solutions. This situation adds to frustration, worry and helplessness as the family unit spirals out of balance. The logical, problem-solving and practical approach from the Baby Body Language perspective that I offer, is often a welcomed relief to parents.

### Sophie - aged three years

Sophie's parents, Thelma and Jack first visited my treatment room very much as a last resort. Thelma turned out to be a natural storyteller and spoke from the heart. As I built up a rapport and quickly gained their trust, they shared more of their family situation, relieved by the sharing of the emotional journey they had experienced to date. It was a journey of one medical emergency after another which had them constantly on the alert. I got the impression that both Thelma and Jack were open to reviewing Sophie's situation from another angle as if they instinctively knew there was something more that could be done for their youngest child.

At their initial consultation in late November 2015, Thelma was cradling their third child, three-year-old Sophie, in her arms as her husband Jack sat next to her on my treatment room sofa. They both looked dazed and exhausted whilst their daughter appeared sickly and limp with her little head lolling to one side. Mum apologised for running late for their appointment as they had been delayed at an open morning at the playgroup that Sophie would be attending after Christmas. My immediate thought was that this poor child would not be in any fit state to start a playgroup in a matter of weeks. Sophie had a nasogastric tube taped to the side of her little cheek, thick discoloured snot ran from her nose, as she coughed weakly and wiped it through her thin head of fine, dry brown hair that lacked lustre or shine. Sophie appeared totally disinterested in her surroundings and content to sit on mum's lap as she didn't appear to have the energy to do anything else.

Mum explained that Sophie had not only been diagnosed with Down's Syndrome but that she had also been diagnosed with a genetic heart and intestinal defects that required immediate surgery shortly after birth during which the greater part of her large intestine was removed. As a consequence she needed daily bowel washes which required both of her parents to do and was becoming more challenging to carry out with age, for both Sophie and her parents. She was also on the waiting list for major heart surgery at Great Ormond Street Children's Hospital (GOSH). Thelma made a comment in passing that Sophie had been hospitalised as an emergency at least once a month since birth. Mum had heard that I specialised in working with children and she was interested in the fact that I practised craniosacral therapy. Although Thelma candidly mentioned that attending was "a long shot" as their expectations for a positive outcome were very low.

### Boosting the immune system

I briefly explained the benefits of craniosacral therapy and how it involved a very light touch of the head and body. Having stoked her parents' interest and got permission to proceed in the usual gentle way, I placed one hand lightly over Sophie's lower back and the other at the front over her lower tummy area. Sophie had a very extended abdomen as she retained a lot of gaseous wind due to the lack of gut motility; her gut was not contracting and stretching optimally due to the loss of most of her large intestines. I explained how my hands were lightly in contact with the back of Sophie's pelvis, my left hand over the sacral area at the tailbone and my right hand over the pubic symphysis at the front as I was cradling her pelvic basket as if giving it dual support whilst facilitating fascial tissue[8] release of the tension she held. I was palpating (or tuning in) to her craniosacral rhythm to gently direct some of the energy and tension in her torso down into her legs and out through her feet to facilitate balance in both her nervous and skeletal systems.

Whilst I calmly and intuitively worked hands-on with Sophie, I used the communication technique of looping back and engaging with mum and dad into sharing the significant and emotionally triggering points of the family's storyline. This was reassuring to Thelma and Jack as they were able to share more of the emotional layers from their perspectives. It is so important and essential for parents to be heard, and to have their feelings and concerns validated. This situation was timely for both Thelma and Jack given that there were occasions in the hospital when, due to their child's dire medical circumstances, they were simply neither heard nor respected by the doctors and nurses involved as they would have been firefighting and dealing with Sophie's emergency situation and the parents were side-lined.

Thelma took the lead and seemed eager to share as the three of them settled into the therapeutic safe space that I was energetically holding for them. Over the session, we deepened the interconnections between each other. Hands-on work is not a

---

[8] *Fascial tissue - A sheet or band of fibrous connective tissue enveloping, separating or binding together muscles, organs and other soft structures of the body.*

separate entity to everything else that might be going on in my treatment room. Sophie's response to therapeutic touch deepened the more her parents settled in the room, released the tension in their bodies, and expanded their breath, as I listened with the intention to both hear and understand them on their level.

Thelma described the shock and worry in the second trimester of her third pregnancy when they learned of Sophie's medical issues, her ongoing future concerns around the delivery, birth and managing a newborn with challenges together with the possibility of some yet unknown issues. She explained how they were juggling working and family life, together with the emotional impact that the regular hospitalisations were having on Sophie's two older siblings.

Continuing to check in with mum and dad's engagement and understanding of what I was doing, I paced Sophie's response to my first aid craniosacral therapy work. Although she appeared outwardly passive she was in fact, very receptive and deeply in tune with my touch. I intuitively readjusted my hands over other fascial tension points that needed releasing and repositioned my hand contact gently and lightly over Sophie's respiratory diaphragm, in the lower chest area above her extended tummy, to help her breathe more easily.

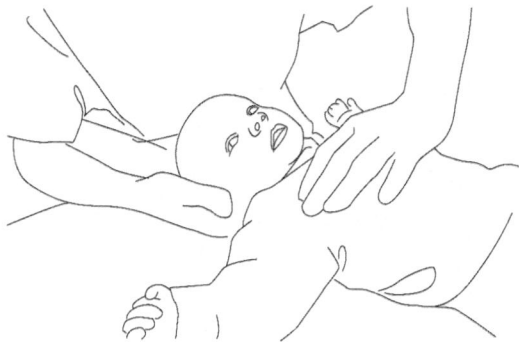

With my left hand hovering over the crown of her head where her cranial bones met, she then subtly softened as the tension in her chest released and she snuggled lovingly into her mum's lap. I tend to work with babies and small children on a parent's lap and often the mums will be able to feel their child become heavier and more relaxed on their lap, as I facilitate subtle releasing of the tissues below my hands.

In summarising my overall assessment and treatment of Sophie, I also recommended that mum massage Sophie's lower and upper back nightly, if they felt that Sophie was up for it. I invited the parents to book a follow-up appointment within the following two weeks. I must admit, I did have my reservations; I was not sure whether I had made a significant enough difference to Sophie on that first visit to convince her parents to return for a follow-up session. Sophie had such complex medical needs; her nervous and immune systems were struggling severely and she was experiencing global neurodevelopmental delay. I parked the thought that Sophie may be well beyond my professional remit.

On the morning that Sophie was due for a second session, I was working from a different treatment room to my usual one, the door of which opened into a short passageway leading to our reception area. I was coming to the end of a deep craniosacral session with an adult, and we were being interrupted by a child knocking on the door and running back and forth in the passageway. My immediate reaction was that of disappointment. I immediately assumed that Sophie's parents had cancelled her appointment at the last minute and that my support staff had scheduled another older child in Sophie's place. Although I had some doubts, I still wanted to have a shot at treating Sophie given that her devoted parents and family needed hope by the bucket loads for their little girl.

When I went out to reception to greet my next client, I was met by a bright little girl with a glint in her eye who was running around the reception and waiting area entertaining the other patients. It was Sophie! Her mum said she simply went from strength to strength each day after the first session and found her "mojo" like she never had before. On reflection, this was the significant turning point for Sophie with Thelma commenting many months later that "she hasn't looked back."

Mum also mentioned that, from that first session, Sophie had not had any unscheduled hospitalisations, when previously they had been monthly. Her response to treatment had made such a huge difference to family life on so many levels. At the times when Sophie would become very sick and was running a temperature, her parents (who both worked full-time) would take turns maintaining a nightly vigil to watch over her. Then, if the situation became critical, they would make an emergency visit to the hospital whilst sorting last-minute childcare for their other two children. This had been the ongoing stressful situation month after month for the previous three years.

Within two years, following her initial session with me, Sophie's health had improved so much that her white blood cell count was low and sufficiently stable for the cardiac surgeon at Great Ormond Street Hospital to proceed with her much-needed heart valve surgery.

## The Family's health and wellbeing

As a therapeutic practitioner, I have observed countless times when a change in the physiological and emotional state is facilitated in one member of a family, others will follow; it is the "drop in the pond" effect where the ripples spread far and wide. The benefits of improving the health and neurodevelopmental progress of a child by enhancing the balance of their nervous system with craniosacral therapy can, in turn, have a significant beneficial effect on those around them. It empowers parents to have the confidence and motivation to explore other ways to benefit their children and family members and to expand the quality and resonance of the family field.

The health and wellbeing of each member of a family living together tends to have an impact on each of the other individuals in some shape or form. In addition, the growth and development of anyone within that family can enable or inspire growth of the others. In Sophie's family's case, it was a pleasure to watch her mum commit to study and qualify as a kinesiologist, several years after their initial consultation. Thelma was motivated by her passion to maintain Sophie's immune system by providing her and all the family with essential nutrition and supplements, healing therapies and a healthy outdoor environment. The journey of caring for a child with complex medical needs has motivated many mums that I have worked with to seek more meaningful, vocational work which has longer-term benefits for both them and their children.

When I invited Thelma and Jack to contribute to this book, Thelma wrote,

*"It is certainly a much better place to be, in control and moving forward with techniques and therapies that we know work rather than leaving it to the sometimes quite hapless plan of the hospital. Of course, we know Sophie would not be here without their surgeries but, on the other hand, we could also say she might not be here if we hadn't moved forward with our own health plan for Sophie."*

Integrating the knowledge that comes with a diagnosis or label can be empowering. For many parents, diagnostic labels help define the problems their children face and allow for greater understanding. Having a name for the condition means the parents can acquire knowledge, seek help and act to better the situation. One parent whose child was diagnosed with autism remarked that,

*"Labelling our child was the best thing we could have done, simply because it changed our children from bizarre and (sometimes) badly behaved to different but (mostly) well-behaved."*

---

**"A medical diagnosis does not have to define nor limit your child's progress. It can help you to understand, seek support and take action to better their situation."**
**Anne Matthews**

---

### Noah, aged three years four months

### The Parents' Story

Lisa and Brendan attended with their son, Noah.

*"Having recently received a diagnosis of autism, we were beside ourselves with worry about what the future held for Noah and where we could turn to get help for him. From the very first appointment, we started to gain knowledge and understanding; an understanding of what our son's day-to-day challenges are, why he does the things that he does and why he finds some day-to-day activities such as walking, talking making eye contact so difficult. Anne's approach was very empathetic and non-judgemental from the outset.*

*"Anne explained some of the reasons for the physical challenges that he faced daily and gave us an understanding of how*

we could try to work with him. One thing that stands out is that Anne was not hung up on our child's diagnosis, explaining that he was very young and for us to start working on the simple tasks to engage and understand how to teach him to regulate and cope with the world around him. In the first few sessions, Anne made us feel very comfortable with very little expectation for Noah to engage with her. This really helped as he needed to build that trust and get to know her.

During the early sessions, we were educated on some interesting information about the cranium, the brain and the central nervous system. This was important as we needed to understand why soft massage could help our son physically as well as being a tool for us to build rapport with him and engage with him.

"At the time, our son was very clingy with me and not so much with dad. Anne explained how this could relate back to feeling safe and content in the womb and to some extent I was still his safe place. We were advised in the first session to massage him softly by rubbing lotion lightly on his lower and upper back which Anne demonstrated to us. We found, after a couple of sessions, that Noah's eye contact was improving and his words were coming.

"Every single session that we went to, we left feeling that not only had we made progress but also we were really starting to understand how to navigate different challenges. The fear we felt as parents started to lessen.

"Anne always reassured us and encouraged us to keep going, to keep working with him. When our son's language started to build, he was able to communicate that he wanted to go and see Anne; he knew that his visits there made him feel better and he looked forward to going.

## Progress and development

*"Our son has gone from a child whose balance was way off, wobbling all over the place, to a child who can climb, run without falling and hop on one leg. From a non-verbal child to a child who can talk (albeit about his interests), communicate his needs most of the time and has started to read some words.*

*"The biggest and most beneficial change in him, we feel, is his ability to better regulate his emotions. He can cope with emotions much better and he has learned his own coping mechanisms. Anne has been excellent at mentoring us to help him to be able to do this, to learn his Baby Body Language and has been an unbelievable support to us as parents.*

*"Our family has benefitted from having support that is always caring, always in touch with how both child and parents are feeling and never judgemental. Taking our child through the doors of Belfast Chiropractic Clinic was the best move we have made to date and we look forward to watching Noah's progress under professional guidance."*

## What was the back story?

When Lisa first attended with Noah and her husband, her nervous system was running on high alert and she was eager to relay every single detail regarding Noah's situation to date. She related several negative experiences with other professionals regarding Noah's care and felt that she was being regarded as an over-anxious older mum and that she was not being heard as an advocate for her non-verbal child.

Lisa was passionate about providing early interventions and creating opportunities for Noah. Brendan, however, mentioned at the initial consultation that his son's resistance and inflexibility to everyday life was such a challenge that he did not expect him to make any significant progress and that they had to find a way to live with that. This was also based on the fact that Noah was disinterested in his dad, with mum being the only person who could manage his outbursts.

Lisa described Noah as a much-wanted and planned baby and mum opted for an elective C-Section, citing her age (38 years old) as the prime reason. She described how Noah had been an unsettled and fussy baby around feeding, had walked at 18 months after crawling on all fours, although he tended to walk on his toes, and had difficulty remaining still whilst standing or sitting. He also had sensory issues, disliking certain sounds, food, clothes and touch.

**In the treatment room**

At the first session, Noah was very active in the room, moving from one thing to another, as mum quietly and calmly talked to him in simple and direct language. Mum would divert his attention from excess physical movement using a range of distraction activities/toys that she would bring to the sessions, such as play dough, fidget toys and dinosaurs which were a big hit at the beginning.

I explained to Lisa that her technique of foreseeing and managing Noah's behaviour was helping him to regulate his nervous system. In fact, it was like helping him to keep a lid on the things that triggered his fight/flight response which, in turn, allowed Noah's nervous system to feel safe. Lisa's approach was necessary and worked well. I explained that, as time went on, Noah would be best supported to learn to do this for himself - namely, to self-regulate, otherwise it could become increasingly more difficult and complex if she and her husband needed to continuously scan for cues and situations that have the potential to trigger Noah's nervous system and to make him feel unsafe. In fact, Noah was showing signs of having a retained Moro Reflex <sup>Moro Reflex@.</sup>

The Moro Reflex develops around the thirteenth week of gestation in the womb. It develops to help protect the baby from danger sensed through the sensory system and to take their first breath of life. When a newborn is startled or receives sensory input like a jarring, sudden light or sound, their arms flail out, the baby quickly takes a deep breath, then curls up crossing both the arms and legs. This is an involuntary reflex that is part of normal development and should disappear between two-four months of age. Because this reflex is triggered by the sensory systems, it can cause an array of problems if it remains longer as a retained reflex.

My approach was to help Noah's parents understand why his system was on continuous high alert and to give them tools to bring his nervous activity level down a notch or two. Practical tools were needed to assist Noah and, in turn, empower both Lisa and Brendan to help their child constructively and with specific purpose rather than from a "firefighting" perspective.

It can be physically and emotionally exhausting for a child, or any person, to be continually triggered to high alert as it depletes both the immune and nervous systems and demands high levels of the stress hormone, cortisol, to help rectify the system. As we also witnessed with Tommy in Chapter Two, children in this mode tend to rely on fast-releasing carbohydrates, such as pasta and bread, to feed their overactive system and they are often described as fussy eaters due to their very restrictive diets to meet their limited nutritional needs.

Parents benefit from being facilitated and guided in relating to and understanding the pre and perinatal (PPN) journey that their child may have had; from being conceived, being emotionally wanted or unwanted and the ups and downs, and doubts, that mum may have had whilst the baby was growing and developing in the womb. Mum's mental state, the level of her emotional resilience, her emotional experiences, her memories around previous pregnancies (wanted, unwanted or unexpected) and her expectations around birthing or previous birthing experiences all contribute to a child's early imprints. These factors directly affect how babies form their first relationships at a time of non-verbal communication as part of their embodied experiences.

It is useful to reflect and consider how a baby was valued and loved as they developed in the womb; how the baby, prenatally, was readily nourished with good nutrition from the umbilical cord; how mum related and connected to her baby in the womb; how mentally healthy mum was and how she was emotionally supported during her pregnancy; how mum dealt with stresses, grief, sadness, joy and excitement during her pregnancy; how mum was looking forward to and preparing for each trimester and for the birth; how mum connected with her baby to explain that the birth may not be as the baby's natural blueprint had intended. A baby in the womb is a conscious, sensitive being who has expectations and their own experiences, as well as relating and connecting with their mum's experience.

Lisa and Brendan embraced this approach, as did Noah. As they were very hands-on and committed, I met them where they needed to be met. I started them off with one daily task. As you will understand from reading about my approach in this book, giving massages is often suggested for a child at bedtime. Noah readily got into the swing of it, lying on his tummy over a pillow after he had a bath and was ready to settle down for the night. This is an ideal time to help a child to regulate their nervous system as he may have been triggered from emotional chaos to emotional exhaustion many times during the day.

Massage helps in so many ways due to the amazing power of touch. It is a portal of connection from parent to child and, as this connection strengthens, parents will also realise that they too benefit from the emotional experience derived from this nightly ritual. A child will feel a discharge of emotional nervous energy as his muscles are gently stretched and their trigger points, or knots, released and the child is encouraged to actively exhale. The child will naturally sense into this subconsciously, and later consciously, as they actively become aware of letting go of their feelings and emotions with the release of the tissues. A child will feel more relaxed and more ready for their NS to slip into sleeping mode. With patience and practice, a child will seek out this evening ritual from a parent who, in turn, will also experience the increasing satisfaction and then delight of being able to settle their child.

To read and interpret some significant aspects of your baby's and child's journey to date will help to empower you as a parent and re-orientate the way in which you interact and connect with your child. As your child's BBL has been formed around their earliest experiences in the womb and at birth, let's avail of this wonderful opportunity to tune in!

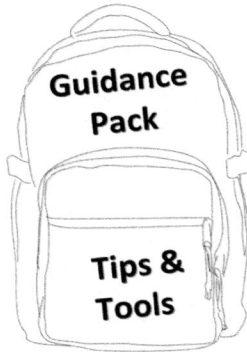

Guidance Pack

Tips & Tools

**"You don't need proof when you have instinct."**

**Awareness**

**Six steps in developing your intuition as a parent**

- Notice your child's breathing rhythm - do they hold their breath when under pressure or shocked?

- Do they have difficulty catching their breath when crying? Or do they tend to sob uncontrollably?

- How do you know they are stressed? Do they kick their feet or push away with their hands? Or shake their head or bang it on a hard surface?

- Does your child need to be held tightly when being comforted? Or do they need their personal space with you close by?

- How does your child interact with their eyes when stressed? Are their eyes closed or searching for you? Do their eyes look alert and shocked or gone?

- What distractions do they respond to, if any?

## Reflections

**In the past ...**

- Has there been a situation when you felt you were not being heard or your point of view was not being considered by a health professional?

- How did you feel at the time?

- Sense into your body - how does it feel now as you recall the event?

- How did your baby or child react when you were in that situation?

- Practise your 1:2 breathing and place your feet on the floor as you record your thoughts in your journal.

# Chapter Four

## From the Baby's Perspective

*"Your child wants to share their wins! Be the first to hear!*
***Anne Matthews***

Developing our understanding and application of Baby Body Language (BBL) requires us to acknowledge the baby's perspective and to reflect as to what that may have been. In learning the birth story and looking at the baby's BBL, we begin to reveal our baby's point of view. As with all humans, their perspective is going to be different from ours.

### Baby Sinead, aged eight weeks

### The Parents' Story

*"Having worked as a GP for 11 years, I assumed I knew a bit about children but it wasn't until I had my daughter that I started the most wonderful, exhausting learning curve! A relative had suggested that we see Anne for some input as our daughter was bothered by very painful wind and I had heard positive reports about craniosacral therapy. The experience turned out to be so much more than "helping her wind"! We learned how she would have experienced pregnancy and the birth process and what we could do to help her find her balance after what is a very big event for a very small person. Since working with Anne, our daughter no longer seems in pain but we have also noted changes in her physical behaviour which demonstrate how she is trying to find her own balance and symmetry.*

*"Many people look forward to the time when their children can start to chat and communicate with them. Anne showed us how a child is constantly communicating with us from the moment they are born and understanding this can help parents develop a real connection with their baby as they read their baby body language. Anne has a very gentle, reassuring and supportive energy that makes both parents and child feel immediately at ease. Her extensive knowledge is obvious and we left feeling empowered to help our baby in a way we did not know we could. Both her father and I now feel we have a much better understanding of our daughter's needs and, indeed, our own in our parenting roles.*

*"I wish all parents were able to avail of her time and I am delighted to recommend both herself and craniosacral therapy to any of my patients. After pregnancy and childbirth being very centred around the mum, working with Anne has been a great way to do something as a family unit. It is fair to say that, every time we leave her room, we have a really positive energy ourselves and we all sleep very well that night!"*

Research evidence collected over the past two decades has shown that infants have capabilities far beyond what they were given credit for in the past, which had been based purely on the extent of their physical development. It was mistakenly assumed that unborn, and even newborn, brains did not yet have the capacity to be aware of their surroundings, to lay down memory or to feel pain. However, research in pre and perinatal (PPN) psychology has shown that newborns and infants are not functioning on a purely vegetative level but rather as complex beings that are sensitive, sensible and capable of observing, learning, feeling and remembering at least from the age of six months post-conception and perhaps earlier.

Pre and perinatal psychology (PPP) and trauma resolution research show us that it is never too late to address the issues that may have been caused by our earliest experiences - babyhood and childhood traumas. Participating in PPN trauma resolution workshops enabled me to resolve the emotional impact of my own early imprints and changed the course of my life's trajectory. Learning of similar resolutions, from the related experiences of many of my co-attendees, has motivated me to offer my clients the opportunity to do likewise. I do this by facilitating the somato emotional release (SER) process of working through the early imprints which have had a negative effect on the development, behaviours and perceptions of the baby attending me.

## Your baby wants to be the first to tell you

In more recent years, I've observed that many young parents are being adversely influenced to the extent that they are over-relying on parenting Apps which map a baby's and child's progress from week to week and month to month within the first three years of a child's life. The information offered that compares a baby's progress to a norm can impact the fragile confidence of some new parents. In fact, parents run the risk of being robbed of developing their own maternal and paternal intuition in these early years when bonding and attachment are critical for the baby and mum dyad.

Observing your baby and being aware and in tune with what the baby is actually telling you in the present moment is key. App-style parenting could be paving the way for a future of "know-it-all" parents who may unwittingly be dismissing their baby or child when they share something that they have done or discovered for the first time. Such a parent may think "I know that because of the App" or worse still, they may voice it aloud to the child. This results in digitally distracted parents repeatedly missing out on sharing the joys and wonderment of their baby's and child's first discoveries and achievements. Reflecting the awe and wonderment of authentically witnessing and sharing in your baby's and child's developmental progress and potential, in the moment, is as important to the developing child as it is to the parent. This is part of the stepping stones in developing and building a healthy child and parent relationship.

One dad, at the beginning of his child's session, watched his very obedient and well-behaved five-year-old daughter stack a set of coloured rings in a haphazard way after I had mischievously suggested that she could stack the rings any way she wanted. On completion, he immediately said, "Now stack them properly" and the little girl immediately did his bidding and her fun, creative stacking went unacknowledged. Or consider the mum who appears to be over shushing her baby whilst pushing a dummy into their mouth and telling them "You're alright." In both cases, these were loving and committed parents on one level who unintentionally dismissed their child in a way that may well impact on their self-confidence and self-esteem. One of my own dear mum's mantras was, "Children should be seen and not heard." Research has shown that our parenting style is influenced by the way in which we were parented. Taking a stance to create change by engaging mutual self-respect in establishing personal boundaries based on compassion, empathy and respect would be a heartening step towards more wholesomely connected family relationships.

### Birth trauma is a taboo subject

> **TABOO**

The one thing that all of us have in common is that we were birthed by our mum. The way in which we were born will have been different but rest assured that it was unique and it has impacted and influenced the person who we are today. Please note that some of the narratives shared around the baby's delivery and birth trauma may be emotionally triggering for you as it may resonate with your history and experiences.

In this book, we will hear more from parents whose children were delivered in various levels of challenging circumstances; from non-assisted vaginal deliveries to those that were induced and manually assisted. We have heard from parents who chose the elective caesarean section option for a variety of personal reasons or who were told by the obstetrician that it was deemed to be safer. Some of our stories are about babies who were delivered as medical emergencies and had life-saving surgery shortly after birth, and some who had additional genetic complications. I advocate sharing our birth stories, not to voice regret or judgement, but as an opportunity to reflect and learn from our own and one another's personal experiences. Let's explore some of the belief systems that have created a taboo around birth trauma. Here are some statements that you may well have heard and believed in the past:

**"Babies don't feel anything during birth"**
**"Babies are born every minute of the day, so it can't be painful"**
**"It's a good thing for babies to cry at birth"**

The notion that babies do not feel pain stems from research studies in the 1940s proposing that newborns did not respond to pinpricks by pulling their limbs away, as an older infant would. A wide range of unproven theories attempted to "explain" that this was due to an immature nervous system or other physical factors. These are some of the fantasies that have been used to support the ongoing belief system that newborns do not feel pain and the universal taboo against acknowledging the truth about birth-related trauma. On the other hand, it is understandable that we find it very difficult to admit that our precious, innocent, vulnerable, pure, adorable newborns may have gone through a brutal process to get here. One of the reasons for this is that we would also need to admit that we, ourselves, went through pain or something traumatic to get here. If that is the case, then let's backtrack:

- What are the emotional, physiological or psychological consequences for us as adults?

- Were we somehow diminished or disabled by our birth?

- What if we were shaped by it and we don't even realise it?

- How can we relate to our birthing experiences to understand our foibles and strengths more?

Understanding the journey that our own newborn baby made helps us to journey back to our own birth experience.

### Practising Empathy

When we understand and acknowledge the pain our newborn has endured to get here, we will take a massive step towards truly knowing who our baby really is. Empathy is a powerful healing force and, when we can accurately see what our babies have come through, we can truly recognise them, know them and bond with them authentically. Only when we do this, is this new incoming soul able to embody its purpose. Without accurate empathy, the new soul in its vulnerable little body feels isolated and disconnected. Like adults, babies need to share their pain and their experience with another person to overcome its consequences. Some of the most ideal births are those where the mum and baby struggle and journey together through the physical pain and the emotional anguish as they transition together to achieve the release, relief and joy that comes at the end; the birth and life on the outside.

# Empathy for our newborn

It can be a challenging reality for a mum to accept and admit to herself that not only was it excruciating for her baby to be born but also that it was her body that was responsible for causing the physical restriction, compression and pain. Many mums do experience pain while giving birth especially if they have a prolonged and difficult labour. This is the enduring labour that most cultures consider in reference to a mum's experience of childbirth. Of course, it is important to acknowledge a mum's experience but it is equally important to have empathy and understanding for the journey and the experience of the tiny, vulnerable baby that is being born.

A mum experiences labour pain as intense contact and pressure against the inside of her large pelvic bones. This compares to the baby's pain which is felt in their thin, vulnerable cranial bones and tissues of the brain and, in fact, down and along their little body as they are compressed against the mum's large pelvic bones. These ongoing compressional forces on the baby in the womb, and mum's hormonal changes in late pregnancy, are further preparing the baby for birth by triggering their nervous system and primitive reflexes to initiate movement and the tricky transition out of the womb. This expectation has been recorded and coded in the baby's blueprint. It's their rite of passage, it's their birthright. Any interruption to the pacing and sequence of this coding translates into shock and trauma if left unacknowledged and unsupported by parents and carers.

The pain, pressure and timing of contractions are interpreted by mum and birth attendants as the labour progresses. As mum orients to the process of delivery, for some babies, the prolonged pressure and pain can feel both defeating and depleting. Our initiation into the world can be intense and painful. We live in societies that choose to ignore or be blissfully unaware of the fact that birth can be traumatic; sometimes it is mild and sometimes severe but it is still present.

I encourage you to pause and note what beliefs you have had around birth; your thoughts on trauma and that it could be a taboo subject. Please know this is not an exercise to catch you out but to allow you to express your thoughts on paper and unburden yourself from belief systems that may be holding you back. For example, one thing that triggers me in relation to this is that, amongst my relatives, there is an immediate preoccupation with the newborn's physical features to decide if the newborn resembles the mum or dad more or an aunt or uncle.

Let us truly see that newborn baby in the moment and acknowledge with compassion and empathy the visible impact that the birthing journey has had on them. In doing so we are recognising that birth trauma does happen. Every baby deserves to be seen and honoured without judgement, loved without expectation and seen accurately for who they are in the moment.

Until we allow ourselves to understand the reality of birth trauma, we will continue to live in a world of denial and accidental blindness. Once we have the courage to name it, own it, embrace it, accept it and heal from it, we can then share it with our children, talk about it to other parents and expand global consciousness of the opportunity to resolve birth traumas.

## What might an ideal birth look like?

In such a birth, a conscious mum is prepared for what birth entails, trusts the process of her body, acknowledges and names the pain of labour and recognises that, when she feels pain, her baby has some awareness of her perception and reaction to that pain. In an ideal birth, a mum will be guided by her contractions and physical discomfort to move her body into the optimal positions to support the descent of her baby within. By doing so, she will be stretching and opening her pelvic basket to facilitate the release and transition of her baby down the birth canal as the baby negotiates turning their head and shoulders towards the opening.

Birthing is an intense, intimate and primal process that involves active participation from both mum and baby as they tune in together. If a mum is supported by loved ones, friends, a trusted midwife or doula in a safe and familiar environment, it influences the birth and dramatically reduces the birth trauma and its adverse impact on the baby.

After the birth, the baby is then seen, held and heard with accurate empathy, meaning they are acknowledged, loved and praised for what they and mum have been through and then celebrated. Baby will feel contained and safe when they can stay connected with the mum during the sacred golden hour immediately after birth and, ideally, as her partner supports the mum with love. This provides a sense of permission and enables the newborn to start releasing the pain and negativity of the birth experience. If babies are loved and listened to in the first few minutes, hours and weeks after birth, they can continue to release the somatic shock that was compressed in their physical systems. In each of these ways, the birth trauma can be released and resolved resulting in much less profound or long-lasting emotional, physiological and psychological effects.

Such an ideal birth is a useful intention to set and to be aware of. However, within the delivery room, there can be several factors that may have an impact on or prevent some parts of the birth story from being fulfilled during or immediately after the birth. Remember, it is never too late to address birth trauma and I will continue to show you how in the remaining chapters of this book.

Nowadays, more mums and their partners have the intention to create a birth environment that acknowledges the baby's needs, meaning that the potential of birth trauma is being consciously considered on some level. It must be acknowledged that currently, ideal births are not the norm partly because of a lack of awareness of the baby as a sentient being.

The fact is that every emotional crisis, every doubt and fear, whether coming from the mum, midwife, partner or obstetrician, will have the tendency to interfere with the birth process and increase the likelihood of trauma at birth. Every medical intervention, including ultrasound and foetal monitoring, chemical inductions and caesarean sections, all of which have become commonplace in antenatal care, increase the probability of trauma associated with pregnancy and birth that can result in long-lasting emotional and psychological effects. Many interventions have become standard protocols rather than life-saving interventions.

### Denise and her three children

### The Parent's Story

*"We attended Anne when my second child was 18 months old, following a recommendation from a work colleague, after 18 months of deprived sleep. We really needed help! We were amazed at what Anne could tell us about our son from just looking at him and it made me realise just how much of an impact time in the womb, and birth itself, can have on how a baby behaves in those early days and months.*

*"For the first time in 18 months, we got a night's sleep! We called Anne our "Life Saver" as this was a new beginning for us as parents, allowing us to enjoy our baby as we understood his needs better. Getting the rest we needed made all the difference! My son continued to attend the clinic fortnightly and then monthly and*

*now, at 12 years of age, he is a much happier child and is aware of when he has discomfort and needs to be rebalanced.*

*"During my third pregnancy, I attended Anne myself as I was now so much more aware of how my unusual heart-shaped uterus, which has two sides instead of being one hollow cavity, made it more difficult for my babies to move around inside as they grew. I wanted to ensure I did all that I could to make them more comfortable inside, to feel good during my pregnancy and to change positions on and off the bed during my labour."*

## Reading BBL

Babies are eager to tell us about their birth trauma. It is what they do, naturally and repeatedly until they are listened to and can finish sharing what they need to share. Then they can finally feel better as they have more room to do what they came here to do - to express the purpose of their souls.

When a baby cries to have their basic needs met, as in being winded or fed, having their nappy/diaper changed, being settled for sleep, or held and comforted, this is referred to as "needs crying." Often parents become confused or frustrated when the crying persists, even when these needs have been met - this is referred to as "memory crying." The baby wants to share their story; they want to be heard and, in fact, more specifically they want to be listened to with empathy because this is a natural healing process for a baby. Crying and moving is healing for babies as it helps them to reset their breathing rhythm. It offers them a feeling of being relieved of their emotional burden and purifies them psychologically and spiritually.

Just like you and me, when we share an emotional story to a true friend who is present for us and hears us in the moment, the baby feels better after they have told their story. Babies will tell their story and share their pain time and time again until they feel they have been heard with empathy and understood. In every sharing, another piece of the trauma that was stuck in the fabric of their being is released.

## Crying is taboo

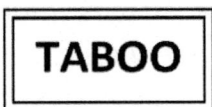

TABOO

It's understandable that parents, for many reasons, want to shush and stop their baby from crying as do many health professionals and crying baby experts. Although this may seem a well-meaning action, have you considered that suppressing a baby from expressing themselves may be adding to their distress? What if I explained that a baby will tend to protest more and more if the need to tell their story is not being met with understanding, compassion and empathy?

Let us reframe our language so that together we can understand, change belief patterns and facilitate our babies in expressing themselves. It is taboo to listen to our baby's cry when they want to tell their story. This specific type of crying is different to the 'needs cry' a baby would make when they need milk, sleep, warmth and comfort, or have their nappy/diaper changed. To allow our babies to move and stretch their bodies intuitively, such as when a baby stiffens their back and throws their head backwards will help them express themselves. A parent who recognises these specific movements will be helping their baby release deep-seated somato emotions. This form of 'memory crying' is an important part of a baby's BBL showing us that they want to be heard with empathy and understanding in the moment.

My clinical experience is that crying which is due to a pain in the baby's tummy caused by an intestinal gas bubble is "present moment" crying and could be referred to as colic when associated with kicking movements of the legs. The baby needs to be burped and comforted but if they continue to cry after the tummy troubles are over, they are letting mum know that something else also requires her attention.

The "memory crying" may well be associated with the trauma that they experienced during the late stages of labour for example. This is when the baby's head may have got stuck deep inside the pelvis and their little head, face and neck were squashed. This could have triggered a shock reaction in the nervous system causing the muscles and tissues of the gut to overreact and go into spasm.

When both "present moment crying" and 'memory crying' are relieved and expressed for a baby, a lot of tummy-related issues will resolve.

Just for the record, it is normal for babies to cry given that they cry for a good, valid reason. It is important that we understand the reason for the crying rather than trying to "fix it" by making the child stop crying to satisfy our own emotional needs as the parent or caregiver. Do remember, a baby is a sentient being who is already aware of what is going on, even in the womb, before they have been delivered or seen in the outside world.

I want to help you to understand that we can learn to distinguish what babies are crying about. A mum who felt traumatised from giving birth can be out of sync with her child and unable to differentiate the types of crying for a number of reasons. Here are some common examples that may resonate with you on an instinctive level or from the parents' stories that have been shared so far:

- A mum may not have felt suitably seen or heard as a result of not having her needs satisfactorily met at a critical point during her pregnancy, delivery, at birth or shortly after. Although these situations may have been addressed by the health staff involved in their best possible way, nonetheless the experiences may have left a negative impact on both mum and baby. These then become unaddressed and unresolved PPN issues which leave a mum feeling disempowered, disconnected and overwhelmed.

- Equally, if the baby's specific needs are not met in the moment during pregnancy or at birth, which could be for various valid reasons, the baby can be left feeling disconnected and unable to resolve their issues.

- The fact is that when the baby was growing and developing in the womb, mum addressed most of his needs and some the baby was able to manage himself. For example, the baby would move his head, limbs and body to get out of a position that was uncomfortable for him. Mum could relate to these positions of discomfort feeling pain under her ribs at the top of her bump, around the front bony part of her pelvis at her pubic joint or is unable to walk without waddling due to pain in her lower back. All of these would be experienced more often in the third trimester when the baby would be more closely packed inside the womb.

- A baby's innate expectation, in transitioning from their intimate life in the womb with mum, is that she will continue to help him address his immediate needs as she had been doing over the previous, 36 to 40 weeks. This realistic expectation has developed in parallel with how his growing needs were met and managed in the womb. A baby expects his mum to be in a similar state of presence and awareness to continue helping him as a newborn. A baby will persist in commanding his mum's attention and assistance to help him shift from the physical discomfort, unpleasant emotion or memory that is leaving him feeling stuck, out of balance and harmony. Babies will cry out, thrash about, be wakeful and unsettled to help mum and other carers read and interpret his BBL and recognise his different types of crying so that they can learn to address his needs. A mum with a new baby needs the continuing support of a caring, dedicated team to help her with the transition from pregnancy to caring for and managing a newborn.

The ideal situation would be that all obstetric and maternity-related and support staff are trained in Pre and Perinatal education including the reading and interpreting of BBL. This would cultivate a more respectful environment of appropriate communication and intentional actions such as being present in the moment to support the sacred sentient being and their mum throughout the process of delivery, birth and aftercare.

A strong focus of my online coaching courses will be to support parents so that they can support their own baby or young child and, in turn, learn to understand and support their developing older child or teenager. In realising and learning to appreciate the journey that their baby made during pregnancy, birth and within the first year of life, they begin to recognise what issues may be unresolved for their child by applying the concepts of reading and interpreting their BBL. A mum's involvement in the healing and recovery process of her child's unresolved issue is critical because, of course, that mum was an active participant in the creation of the experiences and memories for her baby during the pregnancy and the birth. A mum has her experiential narrative which she shares with her baby and the baby also has his.

## Movement patterns in BBL

There are two different types of language in a baby's BBL. The first is volitional which includes "needs crying", such as babbling and cooing sounds; and the second is non-volitional which is associated with "memory crying." Non-volitional movements are part of the baby's pre-verbal broadcast system. These spontaneous movements arise when the baby's body tries to unwind or release an impact, compression or contraction held in the tissue or soma deep inside the body. These "issues in the tissues" may be partly from intense cranial compression (perinatal - during birth) or defensive body contractions (prenatal - in the womb) experienced by the baby which have gelled and solidified and are stored in the soma (body tissue). These issues are wound up in the tissues like a spring which needs to unwind, release and express itself emotionally.

## Storytelling movements

A baby will move and wriggle to unwind these somatic tensions in their body which parents tend to facilitate without realising as they mention how their child prefers to be held this way or that way. The baby's release of sighs, shudders and trembling, after-sobbing gulps, the gripping movements of fingers and toes and the tense joints are part of the random persistent gestures and asymmetrical body postures of a baby's BBL. The baby is conveying and broadcasting the pain or constriction held in their body that needs attention. For example, babies will pedal the air with their legs and feet, with each baby having a different "pedalling" style, to convey the specific story of their umbilical life. Pedalling is a defensive movement a baby learned in the womb to defend against, recruit or recycle what was coming through the umbilical cord. This is part of the non-verbal expression of the baby's prenatal life from conception.

In the pre and peri-natal vocabulary, "conducting" is when babies wave their arms around like an orchestra conductor and, again, every baby has a different style with different levels of tension; hypertonic (high tone) in one moment and then hypotonic (low tone) in another. These movements are not random and, in fact, they tell the story of what happened in the baby's PPN life.

The baby also displays specific gestures referred to as "pointing" during which they point with their fingers, hands or fists against the compressions in their cranium that resulted from the impact of birth. Just to reiterate - pointing is neither non-volitional nor conscious on the part of the baby but instead is a very natural body movement that orients around a body memory from compression or pain. I've summarised the active and fixed BBL and the different types of crying and baby gestures in this BBL diagram. We also see these types of non-conscious movements in adults when their body is talking; for example, pressing on your temporals when you want to focus on something or you are finding it difficult to concentrate; or unconsciously scratching, itching or pulling your ear or your nose, etc. Older children can be observed placing their fingers in their mouth, sucking a pen or making unconscious facial and mouth movements referred to as habits or tics.

### Active and Fixed BBL

BBL can be differentiated further into two types. Active BBL are those I have explained within the storytelling movements above, involving the active movements of a baby's body. The second refers to the static but expressive fixed BBL that involves the somatic expression of the "lie side of the baby" i.e. the side of the body that your baby lay on whilst in the womb. Please view a summary of BBL in the diagram on the next page.

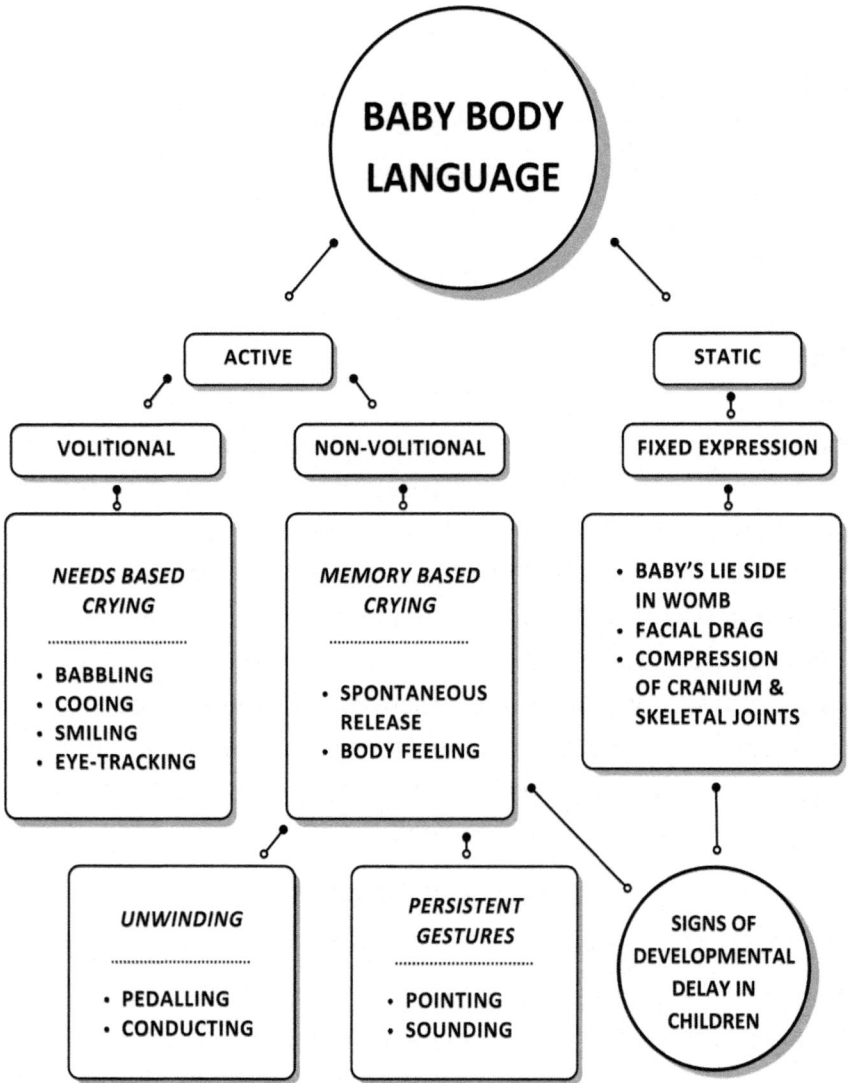

```
                         ┌──────────────────┐
                         │   BABY BODY      │
                         │   LANGUAGE       │
                         └──────────────────┘
            ┌─────────────┘              └─────────────┐
      ┌───────────┐                              ┌───────────┐
      │  ACTIVE   │                              │  STATIC   │
      └───────────┘                              └───────────┘
```

**BABY BODY LANGUAGE**

**ACTIVE**

**STATIC**

**VOLITIONAL**

**NON-VOLITIONAL**

**FIXED EXPRESSION**

*NEEDS BASED CRYING*

.......................

- BABBLING
- COOING
- SMILING
- EYE-TRACKING

*MEMORY BASED CRYING*

.......................

- SPONTANEOUS RELEASE
- BODY FEELING

- BABY'S LIE SIDE IN WOMB
- FACIAL DRAG
- COMPRESSION OF CRANIUM & SKELETAL JOINTS

*UNWINDING*

.......................

- PEDALLING
- CONDUCTING

*PERSISTENT GESTURES*

.......................

- POINTING
- SOUNDING

**SIGNS OF DEVELOPMENTAL DELAY IN CHILDREN**

## Lie-side theory

Let me show you what is meant by the lie-side drag; my intention is to give you a short synopsis of what happens rather than to go into detail about this complex area. The illustration above shows a baby who is deep inside their mum's pelvis prior to being born. The baby is lying with the left side of their head against the mum's most bony part of the lower part of the inner spine, called the lumbosacral promontory. Most babies in the womb will present themselves in this left-sided position as they prepare for their descent into the birth canal. The illustration below indicates the possible drag that the baby may experience as they descend into the mum's pelvis just before the head rotates and is delivered at birth. The line with the arrow shows how the drag is possible as the baby descends into the pelvis. The drag effect is from the left ear and temporal bone, across the left eye and orbit towards the cheek and nose.

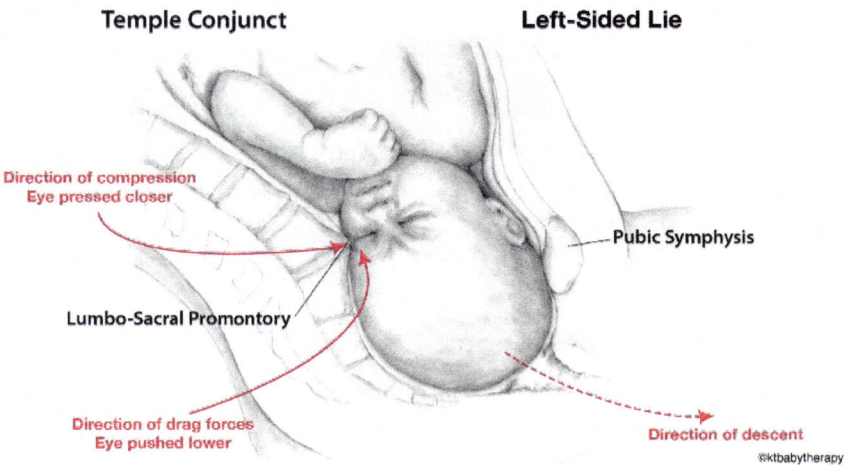

**Temple Conjunct**     **Left-Sided Lie**

Direction of compression
Eye pressed closer

Pubic Symphysis

Lumbo-Sacral Promontory

Direction of drag forces
Eye pushed lower

Direction of descent
©ktbabytherapy

*Illustration courtesy of ktbabytherapy - Karlton Terry*

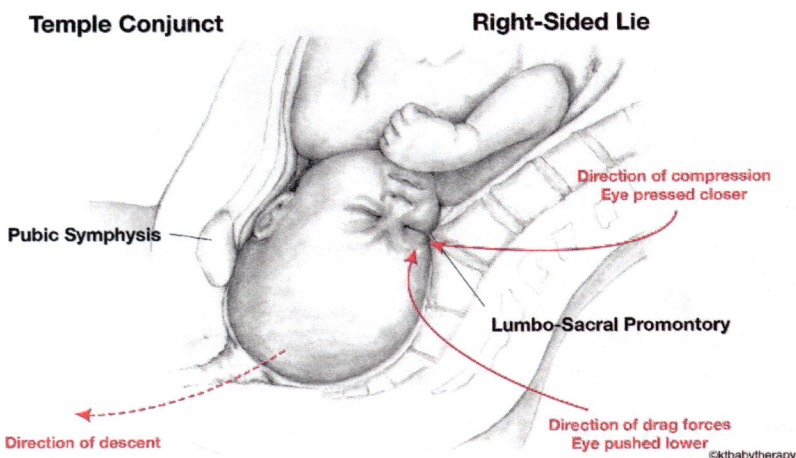

**Temple Conjunct**

**Right-Sided Lie**

Direction of compression
Eye pressed closer

**Pubic Symphysis**

**Lumbo-Sacral Promontory**

Direction of drag forces
Eye pushed lower
©ktbabytherapy

Direction of descent

*Illustration courtesy of ktbabytherapy - Karlton Terry*

To understand your baby's dominant lie-side and how they may have zigzagged down the birth canal is to understand a baby's fundamental somatic-emotional-psychological orientation, meaning that the expressive features of the baby's lie-side are a snapshot of the most difficult and traumatic part of the birth for most babies.

The lie-side expression indicates the inward compression against the baby's cranium and the forces of drag along the side of the cranial bones on the side of the head and into the jaw joint and nose. The newborn baby will often point to it at birth as they touch their cranium with their hand.

As the diameter of a mum's pelvis is narrower than the diameter of the baby's head, the descending baby needs to rotate their head to navigate down and out through the pelvic canal. The fact is that a mum's pelvis and womb are designed to support and give birth to a baby and, in turn, babies are designed to be birthed - it is in their blueprint - that is what a baby is inherently expecting to do!

## BBL expression

So, in summary, delivery and birth are intense experiences for all babies with the impact of the early imprints being recorded as implicit memories in their being. The way in which we, as babies, responded to those memories and the way in which our NS adapted can continue operating unconsciously into our adult life. In turn, our response to these memories will influence the way we perceive the world and ourselves as explained in the Pre & Perinatal Education (PPN Ed) perspectives.

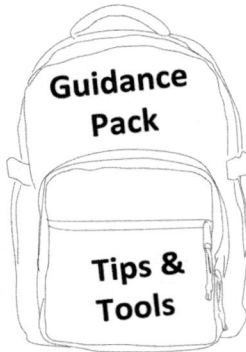

Guidance Pack

Tips & Tools

**"Be in the moment."**

**Awareness**

**Six steps in viewing pregnancy and birth from your baby's perspective:**

- Share your baby's or child's birth story, including their challenges in the first few weeks of life, with their dad or a trusted friend or relative.

- Your baby wants you to share their story.

- They have their own part of the story that only they can tell.

- What could have been different about their birth, if anything?

- How did your baby or child's crying and body movements (their BBL) impact you?

- In what way did you feel best supported by those around you?

**Reflections**

- Reflect on your beliefs around birth and possible birth trauma through journaling your unedited thoughts.

- Sense how you're feeling in this moment as you reflect on the baby's perspective and their BBL, as outlined in this chapter.

- Look into the eyes of your baby with a heartfelt intention and let them know:

**"I see you."**

**"I hear you."**

**"I am here for you."**

**"I want to understand and intuitively connect with you."**

- Know that this is what accurate empathy looks like.
- Take this opportunity to reorientate intuitively with your baby or child with empathy and understanding as you cast aside some of your outdated beliefs.

*There are no right or wrong answers - let's learn and evolve from our reflections.*

# Chapter Five

## Supporting the Newborn

In this chapter, we will look at how to both support the newborn and the family and how to respond to some of the common challenges a newborn baby or new parents may experience. As newborns are sentient beings, they are able to perceive or feel things from birth through their senses of smell, touch, sight, taste and hearing. By looking into the eyes of a newborn, we can allow time for the baby to connect with our eyes, to become aware and sense the resonance of what he knows and feels and what he is trying to tell us. The newborn will understand that,

**"I am being seen."**
**"I am being heard."**
**"I am recognised as the unique soul that I am."**

As a Baby Body Language (BBL) therapist, I am deeply respectful of the reverence of this connection. I invite parents to pause, to practise the intention of being present in the moment and to listen with heartfelt empathy as they gaze in wonderment at their newborn baby. Practising this sacred respect will help the newborn to adapt to the overwhelming and overstimulating world that he has transitioned into. When I work in this way, parents often suddenly realise the depth of connection that I, as an empathetic stranger, can make with their baby and this new awareness normally opens the wealth of opportunity available to them and what is possible when connecting with their own precious baby. I lead the way in order to show, journey with and pace parents as they gain their confidence to learn to "hear" their child above the white noise effect that has resulted from the impact of any negative experiences during delivery and birth.

Supporting a mum and newborn therapeutically and practically, after a challenging birth, offers them both an opportunity to repair the interruption to their sacred connection and allows for the natural stimulation and flow of the love hormone, oxytocin. The release of this love hormone provides the foundation for secure bonding and attachment between the mum and baby. Oxytocin helps the baby's brain become wired with a calm temperament and with the capacity to self-regulate emotional states, meaning their system can be re-wired to go easily from stress to relaxation. The lasting effect of the love connection is then installed and reinforced into the "hard drives" of the baby's brain. Oxytocin is what heals the body. I encourage mums to practise taking a loving pause, an oxytocin break. It is a great habit to practise for your own mental and emotional health and to keep in tune with your baby.

### Differentiating emotions

Developing babies are connected physically, emotionally and psychologically to their mums in the womb. It is important for a mum to be aware of differentiating her emotional experience from that which her baby might be experiencing, both in the womb and after birth. Mums are encouraged to talk to their babies in the womb, to take ownership of their own adult emotions and to let the baby know that an emotion they might be feeling belongs to mum and not to the baby. Although, at birth, mum and baby become physically separated (differentiated), they are still undifferentiated emotionally and psychologically. As new mums, we may not fully appreciate the significance of this transition or have understood it in these terms. The newborn will also need time and support to adapt to the imprint around the intense, and often abrupt, transition of birth. It will take many years, as his nervous system develops and adapts, to become fully separate from his mum. With this knowledge, when a parent or carer refers to their baby or child as "clingy", I guide them to reframe their language and awareness to the perspective of the child and to understand that they may still feel part of mum or rather that mum is part of them.

Struggling with the issue of transitions, and differentiated or undifferentiated states of being, is how and where the roots of disconnect between a mum and baby begin. The mum and baby are deeply linked emotionally and delicately tuned into each other. To your baby, the entire world is you, his mum. Your baby feels everything you feel; he is synchronised with you. If you are upset, tell him what you are feeling and that it is your experience. Help him to differentiate between your and his feelings as he grows. Let him know that the upset, for example, is not about him, even though you realise that he can sense and is aware of your emotion.

## Differentiation helps create healthy boundaries

In the same way that children of divorced parents often initially think that they caused the divorce because the world revolves around them, your baby needs to know that she did not cause or is not responsible for the emotional upset that you are experiencing. It did not happen because of her. Remember, in the womb, your baby is conscious, aware, super-sensitive and intelligent as his brain builds neural connections and lays down memory. This continues once the baby is born and outside of his mum. We can help our newborns by talking gently with this understanding and listening to them with heartfelt empathy by taking those oxytocin breaks and connecting with their eyes.

## Imagine

Let us just *imagine* a few things from the baby's perspective in the womb and as a newborn.

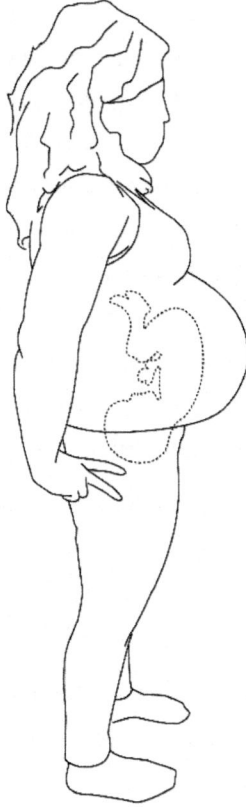

*Imagine* having your own warm pool where you can swim effortlessly and practise your gymnastic moves; pushing off with your feet and exploring with your hands as you move around inside the womb; noticing excitedly the sac becoming more restrictive as you prepare for your big Birth-Day.

*Imagine* having your own pulsating lifeline with its constant nourishment; it feels warm and soft as you hold and play with your cord in your little hands. You can wrap the long stretchy cord around your arms and legs and even your neck! It is fun and reassuring to play with. It is your connection with mum. You learn to squeeze it when you don't like some of the stuff that's coming through, like your mum's stress hormones, and you get intoxicated with the love hormones when mum settles down to talk to you and stroke her tummy and you inside.

*Imagine* the womb as your first school; the place where you learn to move and play; to sense how your mum is feeling and to learn from the way in which she reacts and responds to her changing emotions and feelings.

*Imagine* feeling mum's shock and amazement when she discovered you were in there. She was excited and delighted, or maybe not. Maybe she kept it a secret for a while. Or she may have felt frightened or that the timing wasn't right or even that she couldn't possibly be having a baby or that she might have to get a termination. Then she didn't and you understood.

*Imagine* how the birth was. Imagine how rough and coarse the handling feels to newborns compared with the cushioning effect of the womb and the gentle padded touch of his mum's hand on her tummy.

*Imagine* how intense hunger must feel when you have only ever known constant sustenance and complete satisfaction - automatically on tap.

*Imagine* how lonely a crib must feel when you have only ever experienced the tight, warm and soft embrace of your mum's womb.

*Imagine* how the overwhelming sounds, or the deafening silence and aloneness, must feel when you have only ever heard the soft beating of your mum's heart and the muffled gurgling sounds of her gut.

*Imagine* feeling the hard edges of the world you have just arrived in, compared with the warm place of soft contours and hazy colours within the womb.

*Imagine* how overwhelming the smells on the outside are compared with the lovely smell of your mum's womb and the taste of the amniotic fluid.

*Imagine* how it feels when you have just been born.

### Being born

Ideally, we want babies to move gently into the world outside the womb by providing a quiet and respectful transition with soft sounds and muted colours to help their nervous system adapt at their own pace. All this can be fascinating because they are new. There is no rush about it - they're not going back in!

Let's all have grace and patience for our sentient newborns as they adapt to life in the big, expansive world outside the womb. Their first few months are not a race to be separated from mum and placed in another room as soon as possible. Neither parents nor newborn need to be burdened with expectations of sleeping, feeding and pooping schedules heaped upon them.

To help parents understand the relevance of knowing basic neurodevelopmental facts about their baby (prenate baby) whilst developing in the womb, I would like to refer to some of the everyday references and myths that have influenced an ongoing ignorance around this. The baby in the womb is not "cooking" inside for nine months before being ready to be birthed - like one might think from the idiom "bun in the oven", describing a woman who is pregnant. The birth and first year of life are all part of the fourth trimester which I introduced in the prologue and developed in Chapter Two.

Although emergency caesarean sections are lifesaving for mum and baby, they come with consequences about which parents could be better informed as part of the newborn assessment. Also, when a mum-to-be and partner are informed by the obstetric team that an elective caesarean section is safer for the baby, I often wonder how many are briefed on the benefits of triggering the primitive reflexes in birthing their baby naturally through the vagina. If parents received more information about the impact on neurodevelopment in the birthing process this would help them towards making their informed decision.

Birth is not just a case of "pushing" the baby out of the womb or the birth attendant "pulling" the baby out of the birth canal at a convenient time. The prenate baby has his own in-built triggers and signals that tell him when the time is right to begin the birthing process. He positions himself head down, deep into his mum's pelvis, which coincides with the changes in mum's hormonal system and allows mum to experience the laxity in the ligaments of her pelvic joint and the softening of the muscles, all of which adds the necessary millimetres to the expanding circumference of the birth canal. The prenate baby also obliges, as his delicate cranial bones partially overlap to make the circumference of his head narrower as the gentle compressing of the contractions put pressure on his head, to assist the descent into mum's vagina. The controlled movements of his head, neck, body, arms and legs down the birth canal are managed and triggered by his primitive reflexes. The baby has been practising and perfecting these gymnastic moves throughout the pregnancy in anticipation for the big day.

Mum is familiar with her baby tumbling inside. She can tell the difference between a foot and a head here or a bottom there as she gently rubs her abdomen to let her baby know that she can sense him and is there for him. With each contraction during a natural labour, mum and baby continue to be in sync as they both have been preparing to experience this intense journey together just as their ancestors have done for millennia. It is their biological blueprint.

As a newborn descends head-first into mum's pelvis, it is naturally compressed and pushed rhythmically by the uterine contractions as she gently slides down through the birth canal and out through the stretched opening of the vagina. The repetitive compression and releasing of mum's contractions, controlled by a surge of pain-relieving hormones, also trigger the baby's brain and spinal cord to instruct the primitive reflexes to do their job. The baby responds as the uterine contractions squeeze out the fluids from his lungs, which was necessary for their growth and development and now, in readiness for the newborn to take their first breath, to inflate the lungs and take on a new life-saving role in development.

## What if this journey is interrupted?

When the birth process is interrupted through any interventions, and if the pacing of the compression is too fast, too slow or too prolonged, the bones of the cranium, spine or pelvis can become over compressed and, as if fused, they stay stuck and unable to articulate and move as they should. The delicate and vulnerable cranial bones (plates), which naturally slide over each other to ease compression on the brain, can get stuck and not slide apart at birth as they should. It can feel both intense and shocking for the newborn as the brain wants to decompress, stretch and develop after that period of compression in the birth canal.

When the newborn leaves the cushioning and protection of the womb, followed by the compression and propulsion forces experienced in the birth canal, they are then also met with an overwhelming number of sensory stimuli at birth. It is known that the newborn brain is particularly active in developing and firing off essential communication connections (neurons) just before and immediately after birth. These connections help the newborn to adapt and interpret the overload of sensations from his new environment outside the womb. He has moved from a familiar world of equilibrium to one of relative chaos with lots of sensations that he has not experienced before. Yet the developing brain and nervous system is prepared for the overload on the system. Their world on the outside can vary from being welcoming, exciting and intriguing, to being too loud, too bright and too rough. There may be an overload of smells, tastes and unfamiliar energies surrounding him. Breathing in air and inflating his lungs will be a completely new experience. He may take it in his stride or react defensively to his first gasp but, either way, he's rapidly processing these new experiences to make sense of them.

A newborn needs to have a close physical and emotional connection with mum as he navigates this once in a lifetime experience. In turn, if mum's labour, the delivery and the crawl to the breast has been facilitated at the newborn's pace and without interference, mum will be awash with the hormones of love at birth which sets the scene for optimal bonding and attachment with her baby.

In the course of writing this book, I invited parents to share their story in whichever way suited them best. Some chose to send me an email, others preferred to have a conversation. Here's the editor's transcript from an interview with Suzanne.

## Suzanne, mum of three boys and a girl

## The Parents' Story

Suzanne now believes that it is essential to understand what a baby is telling us, help them to find alignment and, as parents, be supported in the weeks before and after the birth of a baby.

*"I want to pass on the gift of this work to any mum-to-be to avail of before and after the birth of their baby. I want to share about the benefits of learning the tools that Anne teaches every single parent that I've referred to her. In our case, it seemed to be a matter of eventually finding Anne when there seemed no end to the frustrating and worrying journey that we were on. We were the classic case of 'what is my child trying to tell me?' - in that we just didn't know about the work that she did. We had tried many things before discovering the concept that she teaches of reading our children's BBL and the impact that birth can have and how it can interrupt a child's development. This knowledge and awareness have been transformative for all my children. Our eldest was four years old and our second born just a few weeks when we first attended Anne. All our children have now benefited.*

*"Our journey started with our oldest son, Andrew, although I'd like to tell you about Alan first, who is our second child. As a baby, he was very unsettled and appeared to be uncomfortable all the time. We were recommended to Anne who did a head-to-toe inspection of him and, as she was checking him, she inquired as to what happened to him at birth as she suspected this had affected him in some way. Anne showed me the issue Alan had with his shoulder and how it was misaligned which I was surprised at and wondered why I had not noticed it before. After asking permission, she began working with Alan, as he lay on my lap, by gently and lightly touching and holding his arm and the back of his shoulder.*

"Alan began moving his little body in a manner I hadn't seen him do before. He was making these slow and definite movements, with all his body, that he obviously liked and wanted to do. Anne explained that Allan was unwinding the tension he was holding in his body and that these controlled movements he was making were those that a baby would naturally do when being delivered down through the birth canal and out through the vagina. She explained that he was repeating his birthing movements in a way that he wanted to do, in his own rhythm and at his own pace. As his birthing rhythm had been interfered with the first-time round, she guided me to connect with him by becoming still and grounded. She guided me to become aware of my breathing as I touched and held him as instructed and to let him know that I was happy to let him do his thing. It was very touching and emotional to see my baby visibly let go and relax like never before in front of my very eyes from this gentle touching with our hands.

"The work she did in that session, in fact, helped to fix his broken wing, quite literally. We didn't know that Alan's clavicle had been broken during the birth and from the forceps pull, which I know was necessary for his safe delivery. The doctors had told us that he had a shoulder dystocia from the birth but, at his six weeks check, the doctor disclosed that he had a broken clavicle. Thankfully, because his shoulder girdle had been gently aligned and the pressure taken off the collar bone, it was healing.

"My husband, Philip, and I now have a better understanding of the importance of having optimal body alignment and symmetry work and how childbirth can and, indeed, has affected each of our four children in different ways. We have been the beneficiaries of treatment sessions that have helped and empowered us all to do what we can to recognise and address the emotional impact on our physical bodies. I chose to have C-section deliveries with my *younger two children due to the difficult deliveries I had with my first two babies, and I felt that I couldn't go through that again. Before I understood more about birth, I didn't realise that a baby in the womb has specific reflexes which are triggered during labour that helps the baby go down the birth canal and are also stimulated by mum's contractions to be delivered.*

*"That said, I understand now that these reflexes can also be interrupted when you and your baby have had a challenging and traumatic birth as I had with my first two children. Except in our case, we didn't know that with our first child but now I understand why Andrew had the difficulties he had as a baby and a toddler. But I do know from experience that it's never too late to have those reflexes sorted and get your child back on track. I just wish that I had known earlier which is why I tell everyone. After that it's up to them. For my husband and I, knowing and interpreting our children's baby body language issues, and having tools to deal with them and maintain them, has empowered us. It's also created a wonderful bond between us and the kids, we're all really connected as a family.*

*"My children seem to be very aware of when they feel out of balance and will ask us when they can attend Anne again so that she can help them get rid of their "ouchies" which they affectionately call it.*

*"One of the first things that my third baby, Harry ,wanted to do when he was a newborn was to practise these birthing movements as he didn't get the opportunity to do them during his caesarean delivery. This was equally as amazing to watch and reminded me of what Alan had done. To be part of this shift with your baby feels so natural and I felt very emotional and connected as Anne guided me to hold my baby's body and head in a certain way to help him do this unwinding. It was beautiful as he re-birthed*

*himself and then lay on my chest peacefully as I too, made sense of it and Anne quietly and gently explained what had just happened. I believe one hundred percent that more parents should be aware of the importance of these reflexes during the birthing process and particularly when choosing, as I did, to have an elective section.*

"For me, it's like passing on a gift when I share Anne's work with other mums. I just say that the sessions really helped my children and me and then left it for them to decide. Some mums really get it and others don't. That's okay, it's just where they are on their journey, but I know that I've planted a seed!"

The tools that Suzanne refers to are shared within this book and I trust that learning more about each case will help you within your own lives and experiences. With both baby Alan and baby Harry, we can readily see that how we are birthed matters and can and does impact us in various ways physically, emotionally and physiologically. In Alan's case, he was affected physically due to a broken clavicle which, in turn, affected his natural sequence of development. In fact, Suzanne had noticed that, as a newborn, Alan slept better on one side than the other and he tended to fuss when bottle feeding. I would predict he would have had difficulty with rolling from side to side had his shoulder girdle not been realigned. This would have caused an interruption in his developmental sequence to the extent that such a child may revert to commando crawling rather than four-point crawling. One of the myths around this is that it can be seen as cute when a baby commando crawls, particularly a little boy, rather than parents being informed to recognise that the child is adapting to a misalignment issue. As a result, the developing brain is receiving skewed feedback from the child's new patterns of asymmetrical movement and spatial awareness which means their sense of balance and coordination is "off" which, in turn, can delay independent standing and walking.

## Feeding Issues

In managing a newborn's feeding issues, the positioning of the baby's head and body in mum's lap with the upper back snuggled against the crook of her elbow is ideal. From here, mum can facilitate the baby's head nodding movement by placing her hand under the baby's skull so that she is lightly cradling the weight of his little head in the palm of her hand. In doing so, mum will facilitate a release of tension around the back of her baby's head and neck as the baby senses mum's intention and trusts her touch, perception and empathy to read his BBL.

During the first lockdown of the Covid pandemic, I was unable to meet and treat mums and babies on a one-to-one basis. As a result, I conducted some remote work on Telehealth. I demonstrated to mums, with the use of a baby doll, and instructed them on how to facilitate this nodding movement of the newborn's skull to relieve the tension around the back of the head and neck so that the immature jaw joints could function more efficiently in breastfeeding.

## Myth Buster: Newborns are not lazy

A perceived poor sucking technique and tilted head alignment are often observed together in the newborn. If the joints and muscles of the neck and jaw are out of balance, due to being compressed and misaligned during delivery, then the newborn will have difficulty with latching onto the breast. You can spot the asymmetry of the mouth alignment when a baby is yawning.

## Regulation

A newborn baby is so in tune with his mum's feelings that she can help him regulate the expression of his emotions by regulating her feelings. For example, if your baby is crying for what seems to be no reason, notice how you are feeling at that time. You may notice that you are distracted or anxious about something. In order to settle, calm and ground yourself, practise a pause, reflect and take a gentle breath to bring you back into present moment awareness. The fact is that your baby may be responding/reacting to your inner emotional state because he will respond to what is happening in your nervous system just as he did when in the womb. Periodically, throughout the day (especially after a heightened emotional state), pause, reflect and remember to take that oxytocin break. Oxytocin is released when you do anything pleasurable. This is especially important when pregnant and during early infancy as the release of oxytocin helps the baby's brain become wired to a calm temperament level and develop the capacity to self-regulate emotional states, meaning their system gets hardwired to go easily from stress to relaxation. If their environment (their mum) does this, then their body learns how to do this, too.

### Soothers

Dummies, dodies, soothers and pacifiers: to use or not to use is a matter of choice but if you decide to use a soother, do so with the right intention. In my opinion, referring to this baby aid as a dummy can be a dismissive term with the dummy having a lot of negative connotations around how it's used by parents and carers. Instead, I invite you to become aware of and respect a baby's boundaries. With empathetic intention, ask your baby's permission, "Would you like your soother?" Check if your baby needs their soother by offering engaging eye contact and animated facial expression whilst gently touching around the baby's lips with the teat, allowing them time to respond to your question. The baby will indicate if they want their soother by moving their head and lips in the direction to suck on it.

Using this approach means that you are connecting with your baby as you are reassuring them that you want to address their needs. The baby will be reassured that you are not suggesting that the baby should be shushed, be quiet or not call out to seek your attention. We all like to be heard and seen when we have something to share.

Otherwise, your intention could be misread by the baby as mum telling them to "Be quiet, I don't want to hear your anguish." When the baby was in the womb, mum soothed him constantly and automatically which is another reason mum also needs to adapt and learn to read and interpret her own baby's BBL. The situation outside the womb can be overwhelming and confusing for a baby as they can feel uncertain, unsafe and agitated and can perceive a sense of "I'm doing something wrong" or question, "Why is my mum not hearing me?" These feelings and experiences have the potential to fuel a disconnect between the mum/baby dyad.

Many mums can have a negative attitude towards using a soother (which I understand) and it can make them resistant to understanding the reason why their baby might benefit from the sucking effect. A newborn baby's sucking reflex is strong and can be triggered by gently stroking around the outside of their lips. Babies tend to self soothe by sucking on their knuckle, finger or thumb, or on a teat which basically eases the bony connections on the inside of their mouth and jaw that were compressed and got stuck during the birthing process. This need to suckle is effectively helping the baby to relieve the pressure built up from the cranial restriction patterns between the multiple skull plates (or cranial sutures), all of which need to grow and rapidly expand in the first year of life as the brain within develops and expands. In fact, a baby may only need a few suckles to ease their discomfort. This, in turn, can be disheartening for the new mum when she is trying to establish breastfeeding as she may interpret the baby's cue of pulling off as him not wanting milk or worse, not bonding with mum. This action of the baby is a similar situation to the pointing action that a baby will do when repetitively and lightly touching a point on their head with their finger or hand, indicating where it is tender or sensitive for them, as mentioned in the last chapter.

The baby can also run the risk of being overfed if mum repeatedly offers the breast or the bottle when a baby just needs to suckle to relieve pressure. I'm drawn to assessing this situation in my treatment room when I hear a mum lamenting that her baby feeds all the time. This is not a case of a mum being neglectful in any way. In fact, mum may be experiencing an emotional trigger when her baby cries out and she immediately responds by wanting to feed him to ease his pain (and hers, unknowingly). On observing this situation, I guide a mum to pause as she senses the emotion that she is feeling as her baby gets agitated and cries. A mum tends to be very aware of this distracted feeling as her baby commands her attention. I help mums to explore the feeling that is resonating so strongly with them which is often a feeling around fear or guilt. On further guidance, I facilitate a mum in tracking back as to where that feeling may have originated from or when they first felt it.

When a mum relates her narrative, she can become deeply and movingly aware of when and how that feeling arose which gives her the opportunity to express and download the emotion and shock that was associated with it. As she expresses in this way, she is also expressing for her baby as they are both inextricably linked emotionally. As mum takes the lead in this way, she becomes more balanced and grounded to hear her baby and read his cues appropriately. Mum then learns to differentiate between the quality of her baby's crying as she becomes more empowered and confident in wondering if it is "needs crying" or "memory crying" and "what might the emotion be behind the cry?" A mum who achieves this ability to read her baby's BBL is creating a healing opportunity for both by addressing the physical and emotional trauma around the birth. So often, it is taboo to listen to your baby cry to the extent that there is a profitable industry in the baby world, built around this very situation, selling physical aids to medicines. It is normal for babies to cry and to hear our baby in the moment telling their story of shock and distress is a blessing for a parent.

I encourage mums and dads to access a personal place of balance as they become aware of their breath and sense into their growing intuition. The fact is that they may have been knocked off this trajectory by negative aspects of their baby's birth experience or other adverse things that happened during pregnancy, all of which became accumulative and impactful. Helping a mum means facilitating her to hear her own narrative around her pregnancy (and before) and the expectations around her new baby and then, layered onto that, the unhelpful myths from loving but misguided relatives. For example, "All my babies were sleeping through the night by....X days/weeks/months. None of mine were breastfed and they did ok, etc."

The fact is that the newborn is holding the compressional tension resulting from the impact of their delivery on their delicate little cranium, facial bones, jaw and neck joints and the surrounding muscles. A mum's ability to breastfeed her newborn is not only the function of providing milk but also allowing the baby to have essential skin to skin contact, warmth, compassion and reassurance from mum as she addresses the emotional component of the physical insults that the baby had experienced. Guided and supported breastfeeding is a truly natural, healing way for a mum and baby to recover from the effects of their birth trauma. Tension held in the jaw may mean that chewing becomes an additional effort for a baby or child. When faced with a challenge with our child, opening ourselves to a new perspective may feel like we are surrendering or abandoning something that we believed.

It takes power and courage to learn to pace our child and ourselves. In listening to our child, we show willingness to be open to what they are telling us and to help them be seen and heard. In recovering from any type of birth trauma, it is vital to feel and allow what our bodies need, to allow time for closeness and nurturance and to be careful in both our understanding of and the conclusions we reach from our baby's cues and BBL.

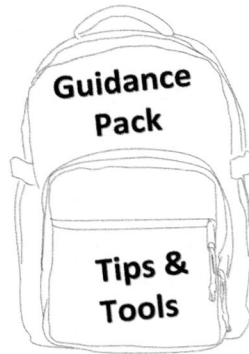

*"Remember – you are doing your best."*

### Awareness

### Six steps to supporting the newborn and mum

- As a mum, indulge yourself in spells of baby gazing!
- Take these much-needed regular oxytocin/love breaks to deepen your connection with your baby.
- Talk to a friend and spend lots of time outdoors.
- Focus on your breath and practice 1:2 breathing as you let go of your tension.
- Recognise and take ownership of your emotions as you release them.
- Gently pace your baby as you practise these tips with self-love, empathy, compassion and patience.

### Reflections

### The thing about babies ...

- Babies are sentient beings who are resilient, loving and want to connect with you.
- Practise your 1:2 breathing with your feet on the floor as you record your thoughts in your journal.

# Chapter Six

## Integrating Therapies for Children

Over the past three decades, my work with children and their parents has evolved as I have added more "strings to my bow" in the form of integrating hands-on and hands-off techniques into my practice. A brief introduction to these therapies and disciplines is shared here to introduce you to an integrative, functional and problem-solving approach to caring for the challenged child. Empowering parents to proactively manage their baby or child at home is a gift that every parent deserves and that can be developed through guidance on using massage techniques, developmental based exercise therapy, reframing everyday language and participating in their own personal self-reflective work. Allow me to guide you through this minefield!

### Prenatal & Perinatal Psychology (PPP)

PPP is the pioneering field of science that explores our earliest experiences, from conception to infancy, from the knowledge that they can leave lifelong marks on our self-image, perceptions, behaviours, relationship patterns and even our health. This science is concerned with exploring the psychology of conception, pregnancy, labour, delivery and the postpartum period together with the intellectual and emotional development of the individual baby in the womb and as a newborn. Ongoing advances in pre- and perinatal psychology are changing the previous established view. As a Pre and Perinatal (PPN) Educator, I weave the understanding of these principles into my work with parents as I guide them in reading and interpreting their baby or child's Baby Body Language (BBL).

The way in which a baby is born is important to their future development. According to 2021 research from the World Health Organisation (WHO), caesarean section use continues to rise globally, accounting for more than one in five (21%) of all childbirths. It further indicated that this number is set to continue increasing over the coming decade, with nearly a third (29%) of all births likely to take place by caesarean section by 2030.

While a caesarean section can be an essential and life-saving surgery, it can put women and babies at unnecessary risk of short- and long-term health problems if performed when there is not a medical need.

Mum, Suzanne, who we met in Chapter Five, explained the reasons why she opted for elective caesareans for two of her four births:

*"I chose to have C-section deliveries with my younger two children due to the difficult deliveries I had with my first two babies, and I felt that I couldn't go through that again. Before I understood more about birth, I did not realise that a baby in the womb has specific reflexes which are triggered during labour that help the baby go down the birth canal and are also stimulated by mum's contractions to be delivered.*

*"That said, I understand now that these reflexes can also be interrupted when you and your baby have had a challenging and traumatic birth. Except in our case, we didn't know that with our first child but now I understand the reasons for the difficulties he had as a baby and a toddler. I also now know from experience that it's never too late to have those reflexes sorted and get your child back on track."*

## BBL concepts

Our earliest feelings, experiences and emotions are embedded in the body during the human journey from conception, and before, as the embryo develops and the foetus forms and grows into the birthing baby and the emerging newborn. Basically, our issues are held in the tissues. As explained in Chapters Four and Five, an understanding of BBL can help us untangle a web of our unconscious experiences and this knowledge can, in turn, help us make better choices. We can re-pattern the adaptive behaviours laid down in our nervous system of past experiences and make conscious decisions to change the ways in which we think and have been programmed to do things. These early imprints are laid down in a baby's nervous system in the non-verbal period of development when the foetus was simply sensing their own experiences in the womb and relating to their mum's emotions.

## Neurodevelopmental therapy

Integrating neurodevelopmental (ND) therapy into my work with children enhanced a therapeutic approach of managing the whole child from different perspectives, rather than viewing a baby or child as separate pieces that are faulty. In doing so, we help children progress neurodevelopmentally and guide parents in working practically with them.

In ND therapy, we consider function to be reflective of neurological organisation - how we are wired in a neurotypical manner. The function or lack of function which we observe in people, particularly those who have been given a diagnosis or label, is rooted in the development of the growing brain and nervous system - neurodevelopment. When there are developmental inefficiencies, we see a lack of function which creates a dysfunction and is described as a symptom. These symptoms reflect neurological disorganisation, referred to as neurodevelopmental delay (NDD) or neuro atypical. Neurological organisation improves with treatment and a child will progress through their natural and expected development stages, resulting in an improvement in the child's neural function. When we facilitate developmental progress, the result is a change in a child's functional ability and a reduction in their symptoms.

Nowadays, there is much hope for the child diagnosed with developmental delay. Firstly, there is a movement towards accepting and honouring the neurodiversity of children. Secondly, a review of scientific literature reveals that the human brain displays plasticity (ability to change), meaning that, with specific stimulation, the function, structure and even chemistry of the brain and central nervous system has the potential for change. Hope lies in the very nature of this untapped capacity of the brain and the central nervous system.

Signs of Neurodevelopmental Delay (NDD) can be observed in a child from three years old, often with a formal medical diagnosis being made when they are a little older. However, it is important to understand that the tell-tale signs of developmental glitches can be noted much earlier than this, even within the child's first year. In my practice, guiding parents in understanding where the interruption to their baby's developmental sequence might have occurred is important. This approach equips parents to be proactive and minimise the impact on the child's physical, sensory and emotional development.

The earlier that appropriate intervention is made, the better for the child's neurodevelopmental progress. The first 1,000 days of life, from conception to two years of age, is a critical phase during which the foundations of a child's development are laid. If a child's body and brain develops within normal parameters then their life chances are improved. Studies have shown that exposure to stressors or adversity during this period can result in a child's development falling behind their peers. Left unaddressed, early adverse experiences such as abuse (physical, sexual, or emotional) or ongoing conflict between parents, can stay with children throughout their lives, can cause harm to them and to others and has the potential to be passed on to the next generation. Further studies have shown that individuals with four or more Adverse Childhood Experiences (ACEs) are at a much greater risk of poor health outcomes compared to individuals with no ACEs. They are also 30 times more likely to attempt suicide. Intervening more actively in the first 1,000 days of a child's life can improve children's health, development and life chances and make society fairer and more prosperous. I have included further resources in the bibliography.

Adverse childhood experiences (ACEs) encompass various forms of physical and emotional abuse, neglect, and household dysfunction experienced in childhood. The harms of ACEs can be long-lasting, affecting people even in their adulthood. ACEs have been linked to premature death as well as to various health conditions, including those of mental disorders. Toxic stress linked to child abuse is related to a number of neurological changes in the structure of the brain and its function.

### Primitive reflexes

A newborn baby is equipped with a set of primitive reflexes that are developed within the womb and designed to ensure immediate responses to this new environment and meet his changing needs upon delivery. These reflexes are also responsible for aiding the alignment and balance of the foetus as it develops in the womb and orientates to descend head first into the birth canal prior to delivery, as seen in the next illustration.

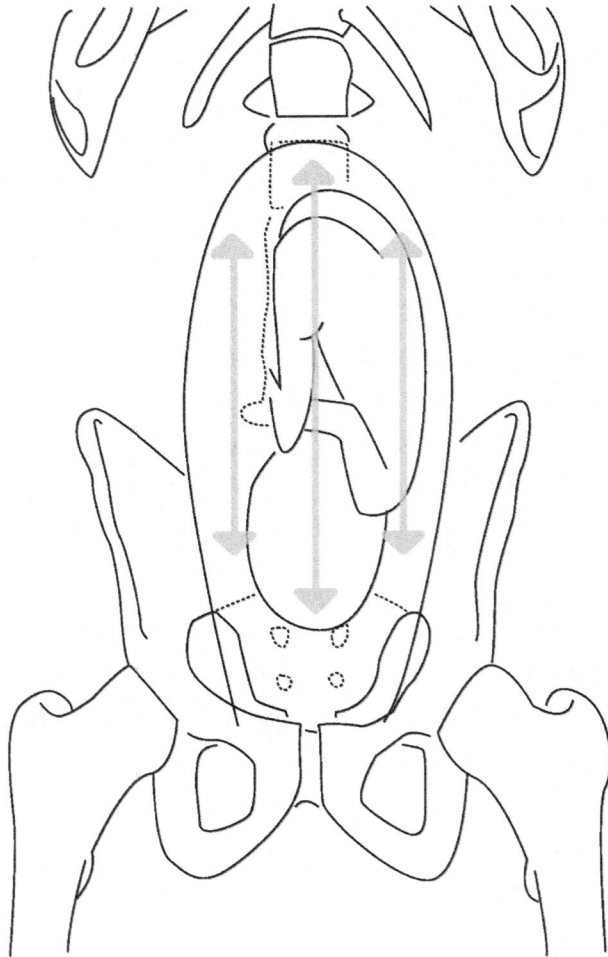

Primitive reflexes are automatic, stereotypical movements which are essential for the baby's survival in the first few weeks of life. They form the rudimentary developmental building blocks for the newborn and older baby as they develop their voluntary skills of movement in order to explore their environment.

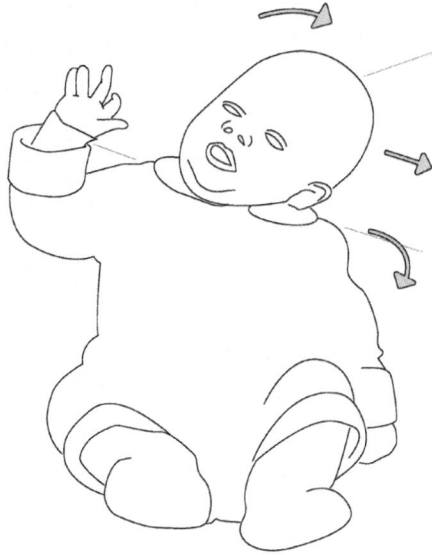

A baby's head and body is compressed and moulded inside the womb and as they descend into the birth canal some will be born with that physical imprint readily shown in their Baby Body Language. In the illustrations, the asymmetries of this baby's head, neck and shoulder alignment are noticeable.

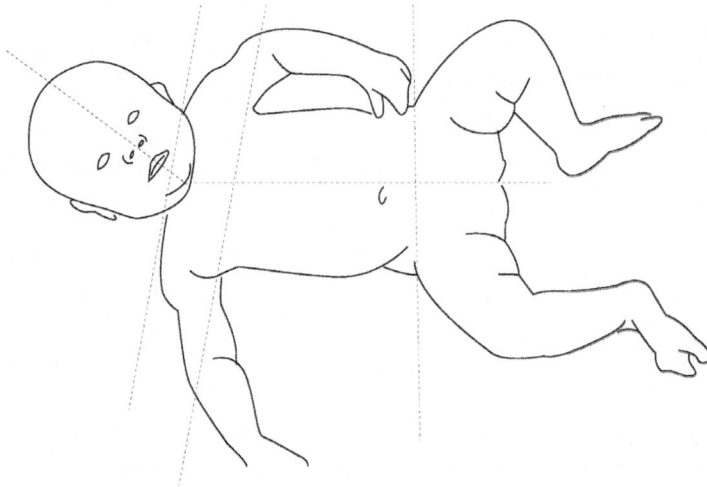

Many of you may be familiar with the Moro Reflex and I supplied an often-cited definition in Chapter Three when discussing Noah's fight/flight behaviour but now we will dive a little deeper.

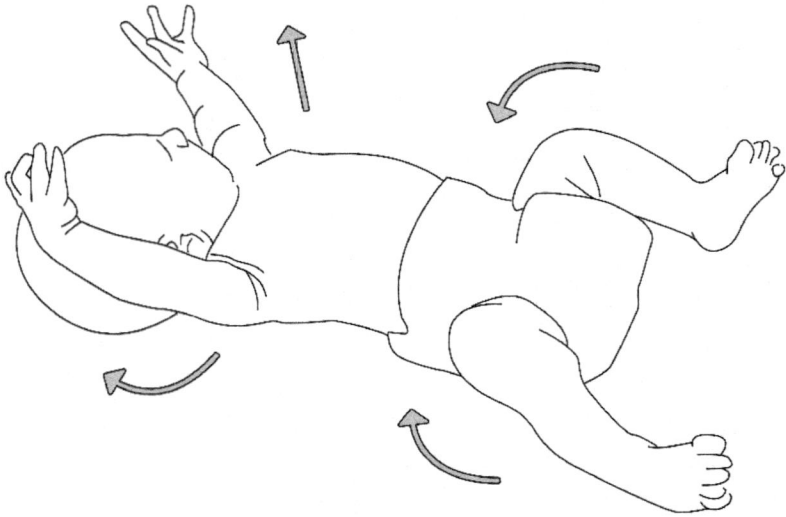

The Moro Reflex is also referred to as the "startle" reflex. We observe it when the baby stretches his arms out to the side when he is alarmed by too much of something and then closes them rapidly, as if clinging on to mum. Another of these primitive reflexes that is thought to assist the baby in moving down the birth canal, is when he will reflexively extend his legs and hips and push his little feet off against the roof of his mum's womb as he actively tunes in with the contractions during labour. A third reflex is designed to help the baby turn his head as he moves into and deep down the birth canal whilst holding one arm straight by his side and the other flexed at the elbow. Later in development, this reflex will also kickstart the baby to creep which prepares them for the more advanced coordinated movement pattern of crawling on all fours and extending their neck and head to look forwards.

These early and typical movements are the building blocks upon which more advanced voluntary movements will develop and be practised by the baby in their first year after birth.

This concept is important because, if the primitive reflexes remain active beyond six to twelve months of life, they are said to be aberrant i.e. they are no longer appropriate and are evidence of a structural weakness or immaturity within the central nervous system of the child. Such a child would not be developing their postural reflexes which are essential for crawling, kneeling, standing and walking proficiently. It impacts the whole child who would also be showing signs of immaturity in other areas of their development. As a parent, we need to appreciate the significance of recognising the neurodevelopmental status of our young baby or child and seek intervention when needed.

A child who has not had optimal triggering of their primitive reflexes nor integrated them fully, will show signs of immaturity; for example, standing knock-kneed or W-shaped kneeling.

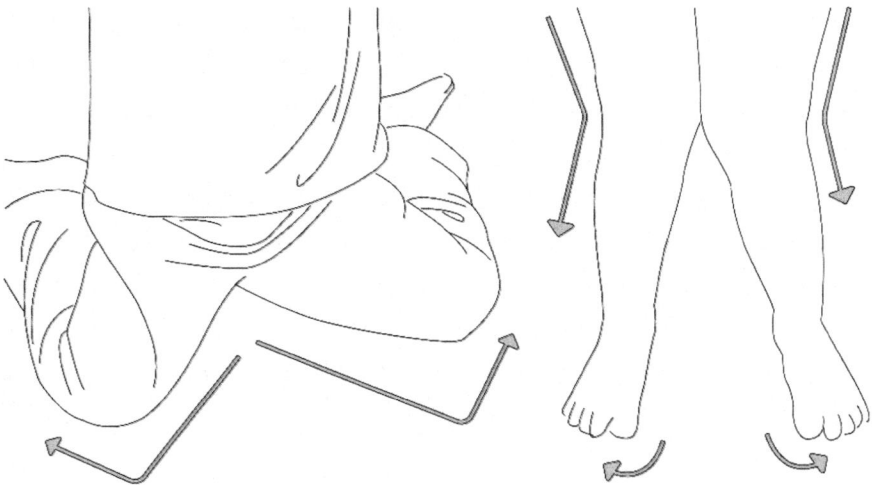

Another example: one mum described her eight-year-old girl as having a toddler with tantrums still active inside. This comment speaks volumes as this child's NS is showing signs of ND delay as her reflexes are probably not fully integrated.

Parents can be side-tracked by the intellectual ability of their child and miss the fact that the child's fundamental equipment of the brain and NS, which is essential for learning, is faulty or inefficient despite their adequate intellectual ability. Aberrant reflex activity is evident when we assess the child's overall developmental profile and his achievement of not only his gross and fine motor (or muscle) coordination but also his sensory perception, cognition and avenues of expression. It may reveal that the acquisition of later skills remains tethered to an earlier stage of development instead of becoming automatic. They will need to be mastered by persistent and conscious effort.

Here's a useful tip for parents - if your child is finding a particular skill too difficult to achieve then review an earlier stage of the development of this skill acquisition as it may need to be broken down further, practised and reinforced. For example, if a child is showing very little interest in straddling, let alone riding, a bicycle when it is age appropriate, I would be curious as to how much crawling that child practised before standing and cruising along furniture. Such a child may also be avoiding rough and tumble floor play. A parent persisting with teaching the child to ride a bike may prove counterproductive. When a child is ready to move onto their next developmental step, they will tend to do it with ease and self-motivation as parents simply facilitate the process, by providing the bicycle for example, and enjoy the wonderment of it all!

# DEVELOPMENT HISTORY

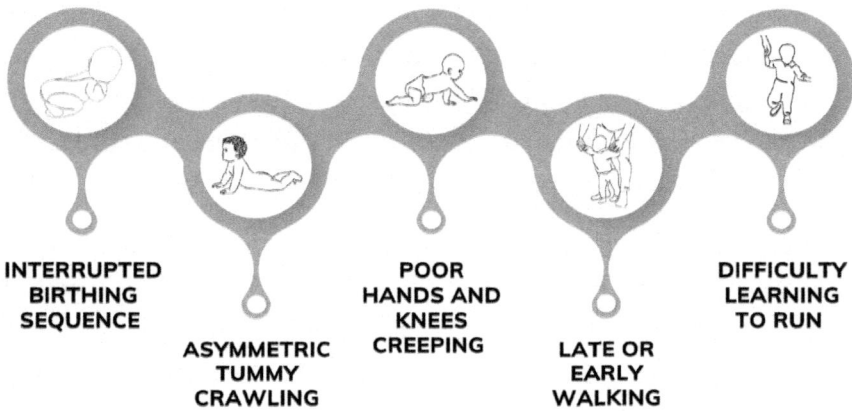

INTERRUPTED
BIRTHING
SEQUENCE

ASYMMETRIC
TUMMY
CRAWLING

POOR
HANDS AND
KNEES
CREEPING

LATE OR
EARLY
WALKING

DIFFICULTY
LEARNING
TO RUN

*Signs of developmental delay are apparent at the critical milestones in a child's developmental history.*

Parents can often be greatly over influenced by the marketing and promotion of infants' and children's toys and products in the belief that a particular product will help to stimulate or enhance their child's development quicker - as if it were a competition to see which baby reached their milestone earliest. As parents and carers, we need to be mindful about how these toys can inhibit a child's natural intuitive and exploratory abilities and confidence in achieving their next developmental step, at their own pace. Some parents are unwittingly being disempowered by such toys and their children are being deprived of their parents' engagement and connection. They believe that these material objects are better stimulators, more competent soothers and more efficient brain developers than them, the child's parents, and that without these products their babies and children will be deprived in some way.

Developmental professionals agree that infants and children are natural learners as per their blueprint and will extract whatever information they need from a warm, loving and supportive environment. The basic security provided by a strong parent-infant bond enables babies and children to reach out to their world and to develop to their full capacity, physically, mentally and spiritually regardless of the challenges with which they may have started life.

A child can experience a wealth of sensory experiences in so many ways - from a mum's eyes, her smile, dad's scent or from the sound of his voice telling a story – all of which provide not only the interesting contrast your baby is looking for but also the loving interaction and feedback. This not only speeds up the myelination (insulation and speed) of the newborn's developing neurons (connections) in his brain, it also sets the scene for him coming into a living, breathing world of wholesome connection.

There is no sweeter music than the sound of a mum singing a lullaby and there will never be a toy that can tell a story the way a real live dad can. There is no substitute for a parent's loving touch as in a massage or a lap upon which to sit to listen to a story.

No vestibular[9] stimulating, mechanical device can substitute a parent's loving touch and movement. As for white noise, nothing can replace the sounds of a heart and breath in synchrony as a baby rests on a parent's chest.

---

[9] The vestibular processing system plays an essential role in the relationship between our body, gravity and the physical world. It provides us with information about where our body is in space. It is responsible for informing us whether our body is stationary or moving, how fast it is moving and in what direction.

## Secure attachments

Research shows that for infants, children and adolescents, developing secure attachments to their parents and adult caregivers is critical for their overall health and wellbeing. Children who are securely attached are more resilient and are better able to manage stressful situations. Secure attachments are particularly critical in unsettled times, as was seen during the Covid pandemic, when other typical support systems, resources and play opportunities with other children were lacking.

Besides love, empathetic teaching and understanding of your child, freedom to move by recognising and facilitating their BBL needs and the freedom to play resulting from that facilitation, are two of the most important gifts parents can give to their child. Both Tommy's and Raghav's parents, from Chapters One and Two, discovered these joyful delights and based their family's activities around them.

## The joy of self-discovery

Children develop and learn most when there's joy in the discovering of a concept or learning how to do an activity. When young children experience movement with this joy, and a sense of daring risk-taking and excitement, they will often burst into peals of laughter. For example, when a young baby masters the movement to roll over, they experience a delight in their achievement and their natural sense of pacing which moves them to the next stage in their developmental sequence. This could be compared with the way in which a gymnast builds up, practises and perfects their final performance piece. These achievements are registered within the NS and give an endorphin boost of happy hormones. A parent who, in the moment, can read and be in awe of their baby's achievements from his perspective, is investing in their child's perception of their self-value and self-worth. This is parenting in the making.

A child's learning begins with exploring his own body. Babies are fascinated by their own body parts and can spend any amount of time intrigued by the movement of their fingers and toes as they realise that these moving objects belong to them. In fact, a child's earliest exploration of their environment is with his mouth. Through the mouth he learns not only about taste and smell but also about size, shape and texture. The mouth is furnished with millions of neural connections to the brain that, each time they are being used, help to "map" sensory and spatial information in the brain. The child who is free to explore with his mouth is also free to experiment with sounds and with cooing, babbling and imitation which are the early stages of speech.

Movement and vestibular stimulation are experienced as joy. Through movement, a baby can explore the environment and express his emotions. Posture, muscle tone and facial expression will alter as his emotional state changes and, sometimes, toddlers will utilise an earlier reflex to express their anger by protest and let you know what they do not want to do. For example, when your toddler doesn't want to be placed into a baby car seat his body goes rigid as the child accesses an extension reflex that was developed in the womb (the Tonic Labyrinths Reflex) which makes it seemingly impossible to bend his body in the middle. As his anger and frustration increase, he will often jerk his head backwards and forwards, strengthening the effect of the reflex and simultaneously working his way into a full-blown emotional download or tantrum. We could view this as the child trying to get their own way or we could be curious to know if the child is physically uncomfortable and is being triggered by the anticipation of being forced back into this old foetal-shaped position.

Although modern baby equipment, like moulded baby seats, may be viewed as a great asset and a safety standard set by law, they can interrupt a child's natural ND progress and become a source of miscommunication between baby and parent. A mum's womb can be viewed as the child's first school and play area with floor play as the child's second. Floor play is not simply leaving your child alone surrounded by colourful and musical activity centres. Time spent with your newborn lying lengthwise on your lap, as you both make eye contact and read each other's facial expressions, is part of the progression to floor play and tummy time. In this way, the baby discovers their own natural sequence of movement as mum paces and facilitates their early progress from the rebirthing movements of play to head turning and body rolling onto their tummy. These movements cannot be explored or achieved adequately from the confines of a baby seat.

Head control is developed as a baby discovers how to roll over onto their tummy where they perfect the skill as they develop control over the postural muscles of their back and neck to look up and around the room. Developmental movements of the baby's individual limbs follow and coincide with the child becoming more spatially aware of the concepts of front and back, side to side and top and bottom. These stages prepare the child for learning to creep on their tummy as they transition to the fully coordinated four-point crawl on hands and knees with head up and looking forwards.

In order to learn to sit up, a baby must pass through these various stages of motor development of their own volition. Firstly, he achieves control over posture and mastery of balance as each stage herald's integration of the nervous system. If a parent or carer repeatedly places the baby in a sitting position without adequate back and tummy time, that child cannot progress through their necessary developmental stages spontaneously. The flip side to this is that the child may be inhibited from acquiring a risk-taking and "I can do" mentality. In the older child, this translates into a fear of falling, lacking physical ability and emotional confidence that would be age-appropriate.

It has been proposed that, for adequate development, a child needs to crawl a mile to fully integrate their early developmental stages in their brain - of course not in one go! The importance of the four-point crawl cannot be emphasised enough as it lays the groundwork for sitting, standing and walking but the absence of adequate crawling is related to developmental and behavioural issues in older children with, for example, dyslexic and dyspraxic tendencies. Although there seems to be a lot of overlap between the two, dyslexia is used to describe a learning difficulty to read write and spell whereas dyspraxia is the term used to describe a difficulty in motor coordination skills.

Rough and tumble play is the direct result of spontaneous neural urges within the brain and suggests that it is during play that various neuronal growth factors are recruited. Studies have shown that animals are especially prone to behave in flexible and creative ways and it is thought that games that allow for "rough housing" help in the development of social skills and allow for behaviour change. In short, this type of play affords an opportunity to prime the limbic system - which is the part of the brain largely responsible for our emotions - it is especially important because it has many connections to the forebrain which is also heavily involved in impulse control and behaviour.

Most parents want to protect their children from the dangers of the outside world but sometimes this can prevent them from developing the very skills they need to survive. We learn balance by falling over and then developing strategies to prevent ourselves from falling again. Discovering the delights and joy of climbing (and falling) helps a child to focus, evaluate risks and discover their growing inner sense of independence by doing, failing and achieving.

In this sense, being exposed to failures is one of life's most important teachers as it engages a child to learn from their experiences. Learning to persist in discovering new ways of doing things at their own pace will give a child personal satisfaction and the building blocks to success. Parents who allow their children to test out their environment, within safe boundaries, help children to grow by allowing them the opportunity to learn from experience.

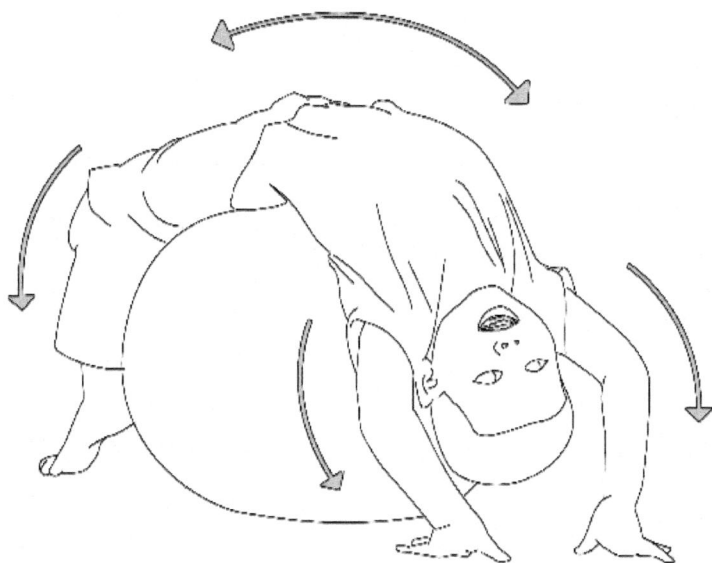

**"Experience is essential food for brain development."**
**Anne Matthews**

## Penny and son Jacob

## The Parent's Story

"I first took my son, Jacob, to Dr Anne when he was nine years old. He was diagnosed with Developmental Coordination Disorder (DCD), Asperger's Spectrum Disorder (ASD) and dyslexia and struggled with coordination and his emotions, having meltdowns daily. He very much avoided sports at school and had low confidence in his academic ability.

"I had attended Dr Anne's Baby Body Language talk and could really see how my son's difficult birth (back-to-back) had impacted him and how his inability to crawl as an infant all contributed to his current behaviour. I could relate to his central nervous system being immature and he had retained infant reflexes which were the cause of his poor motor skills – such as poor pencil grasp and not being able to catch a ball.

"Parents often blame themselves for the way their children are and wonder if they had done something wrong, so it was useful knowing some of the science behind the behaviour.

"Whilst all previous health professionals we attended talked over the child and just seemed interested in placing a label on my child rather than offering strategies to support him and our family in everyday life and in the future, Anne's approach was totally the opposite.

"Firstly, she told me a diagnosis can be a great way of accessing essential help for Jacob as he goes through school but stressed how he doesn't have to be identified by it and there was lots of room for ongoing progress. But what makes Anne stand out from all other health professionals is the way she makes the child feel like they are the most important person in the room – getting down to their eye level to talk to them and explain, in an age-appropriate manner and with the help of a skeleton and model of the brain, what is happening with their bodies and what she is going to do.

"Jacob has a particular interest in tractors and had brought a toy one with him to the first appointment. She used this tractor and its parts to relate to Jacob's body and explained everything in a way which interested him and made it more understandable. I remember remarking to Anne after our first appointment that he spoke to her more than any other health professional in the past.

"As well as making chiropractic adjustments and gentle craniosacral therapy, Anne recommended a number of different exercises for my son over the course of his treatment journey. These included a sea anemone exercise which challenged him to cross his midline; alternate foot climbing up and down the centre of stairs without holding onto the guard rail and a pencil push-up exercise. This involved a pencil being held directly in front of him, at arm's length. The pencil was then drawn slowly towards his nose, and he had to keep focus on it. With the exercises, Anne was keen to keep an eye on progress between appointments and having videos of my son doing them emailed to her. It was useful to get her feedback and make adjustments accordingly.

"It was remarkable to see his progress in stair climbing. Before he would always have clung to the railing and still tripped. Initially he used the same lead leg and when doing the exercises he would veer to the left side of the stairs, even bumping into the wall. Anne commented that using alternate feet climbing the stairs would help him build up his quads and hamstring strength and coordination and soon, whilst he remained slow and cautious, he was no longer afraid of stairs and no longer looked for a guard rail to hold onto.

"Now 11 years and transferring to secondary school, my son is noticeably more grounded, mature, and less anxious. Yes, he still has some meltdowns, but these are only once every couple of months, rather than multiple daily occurrences.

"Whilst Jacob still has difficulties with reading at school, he has really progressed over the past two years in other areas and even won a cup for numeracy at the end of primary school. He also went from not partaking in football to being a member of the school football team – another experience that has filled him with confidence and something I never thought he could ever achieve.

"Anne's approach is very much about educating both the child and parent in order for them to maintain a sense of balance and control and reduce the need for her intervention. With my son his ongoing tools are to draw awareness to areas in his body which don't feel right, such as tight muscles, and asking mum or dad to massage them and also teaching him how to regulate his breathing.

"As parents, we benefitted from acquiring the resources and tools to help our child, such as where best to massage their child in order to help them let go of tension. Anne is also very aware of a parent's own needs and is forthcoming in offering advice and signposting them to help for their own mind and bodies, stressing how a child can intuitively sense if their parent is stressed or anxious and therefore by helping yourself, you are also helping your children."

## Craniosacral Therapy

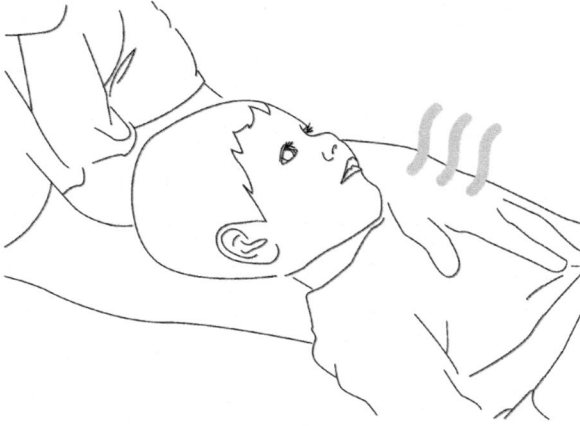

Craniosacral Therapy (CST) is an effective and gentle way of working hands-on to assist the body's natural capacity to heal and self-repair. As Craniosacral Therapists, we are trained to feel the subtle motion in the body and notice where there are areas of restrictions and tightness. We use light and gentle touch (palpation) on the body, around the spine and back of head, or around the chest and abdominal area or the limbs. We can palpate, or detect, tensions, lack of flow and energy blocks in the child's body and facilitate the child to release them in a supported and comfortable way.

In fact, Craniosacral Therapy supports the body's innate ability to balance, restore and heal itself, as well as helping to reduce stressors in the system and build life energy.

Parents will often seek out the services of a CST for their babies following issues associated with difficult or challenging births. As therapists, we use our hands to "listen" to the body in much the same way that a counsellor might listen to your words. The body then responds to this sensitive touch by beginning to "listen" to itself. Reducing unwanted tension and fear within the body, caused by blocks in the system, enables the baby to settle into calmness and helps them get back on their normal developmental path with an innate confidence and self-assurance.

When watching someone do CST, it may look as if nothing is happening as the work is very subtle. Sometimes, a mum will notice the infant's head, trunk or limbs move in my hands whilst I support the body as the infant "unwinds" tension in their own time and under their own power. Sometimes, babies "tell their story" during the process by whimpering, crying intermittently, babbling or spontaneously taking a deep breath and falling asleep. The reassuring presence of the therapist and parents close by gives the baby's NS the confidence to settle and to converse in this way with us. If the baby's agitation appears to escalate, I pace the baby and inquire of mum as to how she is feeling in the moment. I offer her the opportunity to make contact or to speak to her baby and to share the emotion that has arisen for her. She is relating these on a level that is on the behalf of the baby as it's usually relevant to his agitation and he wants to express it as mum listens with love and empathy. Mostly, the therapy is carried out whilst the baby or child is sitting or lying on mum's lap or chest or when nursing at the breast or bottle.

It is not within the scope of this book to explain craniosacral therapy in depth; it is enough to say that in working with newborns, babies and children, craniosacral therapy (CST) has been an invaluable technique in my practice for the past 22 years.

One mum related how her eight-year-old son described the lovely, relaxed way he felt after a CST session with me.

**"It felt like my hair was melting into my head."**

# Chiropractic

*"Chiropractors look at the underlying issues, instead of just treating the surface symptoms."*
**Summit Chiropractic**

Qualifying as a chiropractor was one of the most rewarding achievements of my life. My four-year chiropractic training followed on from a physiotherapy degree as I wanted to hone my palpatory, hands-on skills and read the mechanics of the body in a more functional manner.

Chiropractors use the manual techniques that take the understanding of anatomy, physiology and palpation of the human body to another level. Specific manual techniques employed by chiropractors will involve an understanding of the joint's character and mobility and will apply specific mobilising and adjusting techniques to normalise motion and restore alignment of the joints. We also address the issues of the soft tissues (the muscles, ligaments, and fascia).

One of the most basic concepts in chiropractic is that dysfunction in the spinal joints can lead to dysfunction within the nervous system. Since the nervous system controls and coordinates all the systems of the body, spinal dysfunction can have wide-ranging effects on the body's health.

Chiropractors are trained to evaluate and make skilled corrective adjustments to relieve spinal and pelvic joint dysfunction and to release the associated postural muscle imbalances.

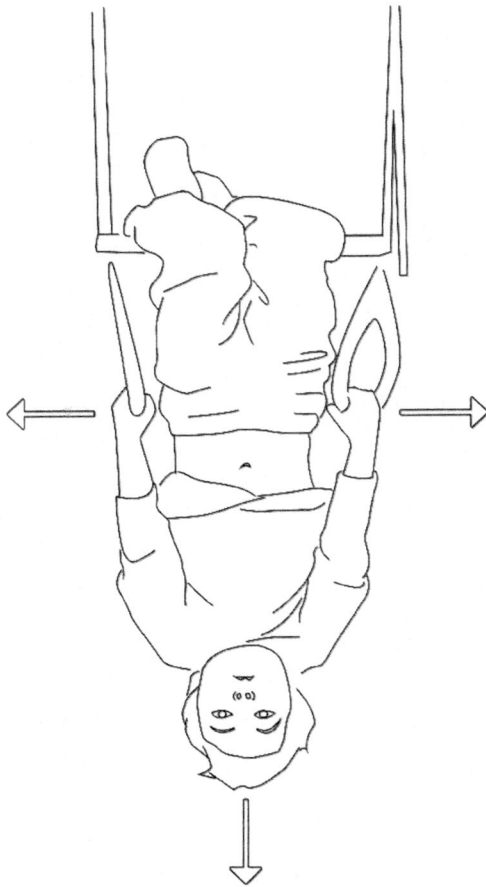

A child encounters many physical stresses and strains during their growing years. The earliest challenge a growing spine may face is in how the developing baby is supported in the womb as he adapts to the mechanical alignment, flexibility and movement of his mum's spinal and pelvic joints and the maintenance of her core muscle balance during her pregnancy. Foetal positioning in the womb is mostly dictated by the space in which the baby must move.

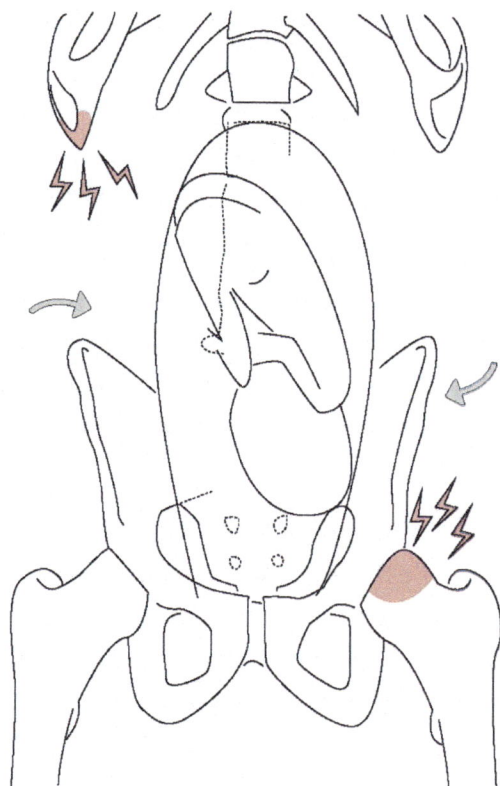

Restrictive postural positions such as prolonged sitting or standing are not ideal for either mum or baby. Common complaints during pregnancy are often the persistent pains experienced under the ribs on the right; heartburn-like pain and discomfort into the groin and around the hip areas as indicated in the illustration above. The baby in the womb needs to stretch and move to practise his primitive reflex movements in preparation for going head down towards the birth canal. The baby is also influenced by his mum's emotions in relation to her expectations around the birth and will position himself accordingly.

In my clinical experience, when assessing the reasons for a baby presenting in a breech position late in pregnancy, the emotional concerns of a mum around the delivery need to be considered together with any past traumatic experiences. The compressional effects on the baby's spine, pelvis and cranium are impacted because of the non-optimal foetal positioning in the womb together with the mechanical and emotional effects of the labour, as mentioned earlier in this book.

The cause of many newborn health complaints such as colic, reflux, breastfeeding difficulties, sleep disturbances and recurrent head colds can often be traced to nervous system irritation caused by spinal and cranial misalignments which place additional stress on the immune system.

Since significant spinal trauma can occur at or prior to birth, many parents elect to have their newborn assessed. Developmental milestones such as learning to hold up the head, sitting upright, crawling and walking are all activities that are affected by spinal misalignment, all of which can be assessed by a chiropractor specialising in children's health. Additionally, falls, sports injuries, playground bumps, heavy school bags and prolonged sitting in the classroom can contribute adversely to the physical stresses of the growing child's spine and nervous system.

It is important to inquire of all practitioners and therapists whether they have paediatric training and experience and if their techniques or methods are modifiable for infants. For example, although paediatrics should be a part of every medical physician's curriculum, the time allocated to this subject tends to be limited. It is also important that you work with a chiropractor (or osteopath) who also understands the mechanics of breastfeeding and is comfortable supporting and working with mums and infants who want to breastfeed.

Here is the feedback from a mum who sought chiropractic care during her pregnancy and had an eureka moment around PPN work and the benefits of craniosacral therapy when her baby was born.

## Baby Cora

## The Parents' Story

*"Throughout my pregnancy with my daughter, I had regular Chiropractic and Craniosacral therapy sessions. I found the CST relaxing and, although I didn't fully understand the therapy, I felt the benefits of relaxation. Once my daughter was born, which was an amazing experience, I really struggled. My preconceived ideas of breastfeeding and the reality were worlds apart. As can be the case, the maternity unit was full and hectic, the lactation consultant unfortunately wasn't the helpful support I'd hoped for, and I mostly had to figure things out for myself. My daughter could latch okay(ish) on one side but not the other and this resulted in a distressed screaming baby. Once home, I tried different positions which helped a little, but I had to express one breast and bottle feed the milk. My partner and I were exhausted. The thought of this being reality for the next six months was overwhelming. My nipples bled, my daughter was unsettled, and I was anxious.*

*"Thankfully, when we attended Anne, it coincided with a time when my daughter was needing to be breastfed. Anne could see there was some hesitance and difficulty around feeding. Anne asked me to observe my daughter whilst attempting to get a latch. My daughter kept tapping the same point of her face. It was a light bulb moment "Here mum, it's sore here." Of course, once Anne explained, her jaw and the right side of her face had been compressed so opening her jaw was painful, making latching impossible.*

*"Anne used CST and guided me to release my daughter and how to support her with light gentle massage and contact. Within an hour, my daughter was latching and feeding well and, within a day, she was feeding like she'd never had an issue. Her unsettledness and my anxiety were suddenly a distant memory. I felt confident in my abilities as a mum and that we'd be able to continue with breastfeeding until my daughter called time, which was when she self-weaned at two and a half years old. I'm so thankful for Anne's expertise; she understood the cues from my five-day-old daughter; she didn't "fix" her but helped guide me to understand what I could do to help.*

*"We have since attended Anne for appointments which always seem to make a shift in my daughter's development. For example, my daughter creeped on her tummy and didn't especially enjoy tummy time. After visiting Anne, the next day four-point crawling was achieved. I hadn't realised what was inhibiting my daughter's ability to go on all fours. Anne, of course, could see the underlying issue and, with light gentle treatment, helped my daughter to shift.*

*"My daughter, now 6 years old, enjoys her treatment sessions; she says she feels relaxed on the drive home, and she always sleeps well after her sessions. Anne's approach to care is very much on the child's level and she intuitively follows their cues. One session, Anne was working on the side of my daughter's head whilst she played on the floor. My daughter was very focused playing but went still and you could sense she was having a big release; there was reddening of her skin and sweating - this was around the area that she had tapped at five days old - and then my daughter gently took hold of Anne's hand and moved it away. Anne didn't force anything; she respected my daughter's communication that she'd had enough and revisited another time. This is an area I*

work on too with Anne's guidance; I find my daughter will grind her teeth in her sleep and I gently massage this area and she stops grinding.

"The combination of Chiropractic care and CST has meant my daughter's pelvis and spine alignment has always been optimal, which has resulted in a well-balanced active child who is confident in her body and its capabilities. Anne has helped her gain a sense of where she feels her emotions in her body and can describe where she holds her worry or relaxation and asks for a massage or relaxing bath when she feels she needs them.

"I too have benefited from Anne's care; the postpartum pelvis treatment and releasing the tension I held in my upper back and neck was a huge help in being able to feed comfortably and as part of my after-birth recovery. I'm not sure where either of us would be without the care or guidance."

### The jaw joints

In newborns, the jaw joints are not fully developed because the lower part of the jaw is at a less developed stage to allow for overlapping of the cranial plates and compression of the facial bones during the descent into the birth canal. In the first year of life, there is a huge amount of growth and expansion as the skull, facial bones and jaw joints realign and assist the growth and development of the brain within. Assessing the jaw joints of a newborn with feeding issues by directing or pushing their mouth onto the breast is not ideal as it may be inadvertently causing more issues and even pain around that area. The techniques of a chiropractor and craniosacral Therapist are preferable in the management of such feeding issues related to the mechanical misalignment and compression of the cranium and jaw joint function.

## Massage - the gift of touch

Massage is an ancient practice used primarily in many traditional cultures because touch is considered healthful, both physically and spiritually. Infant massage is a wonderful way to gently nurture and spend time with your baby. It encourages interaction and connection between the mum and baby dyad whilst helping the baby to relax, reduces crying and aids sleep.

*"Being touched and caressed,*

*Being massaged is food for the infant.*

*Food as necessary as minerals, vitamins and proteins."*

*Dr Frederick Leboyer*

Infant massage can connect you deeply with your baby. It helps you to understand your baby's unique non-verbal language - his BBL - and guides you to respond with love and respectful empathetic listening.

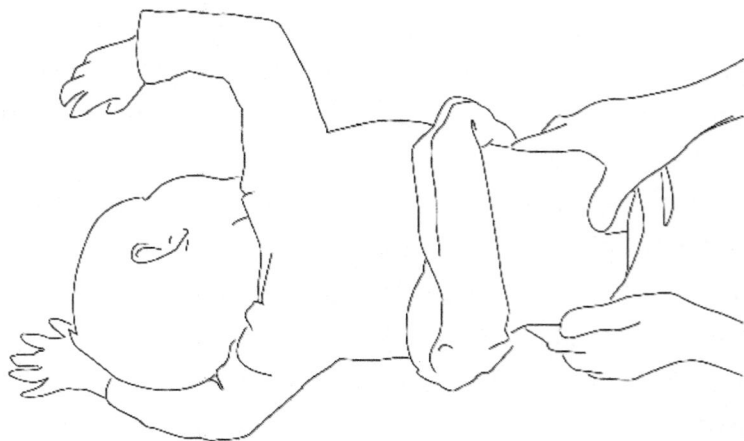

Physical massage acts in much the same way in humans as licking and keeping in close contact does in animals. Animals that are not licked, cared for, caressed or are not allowed to cling in infancy will tend to grow up scrawny and more vulnerable to stress. Licking, as with massage, serves to stimulate the physiological systems and to bond the young with the mum. One reason you don't see a colicky kitten is that a mum cat can spend fifty percent of her time licking her babies. It has been suggested that a human mum's extended labour helps make up for the lack of postpartum licking as seen in other mammals. For the human infant, the compressional effect of the contractions in labour provides some of the same type of skin stimulation preparation for the functioning of his internal systems as early licking of the newborn does for other mammals.

Similar studies have shown that premature human babies, who were held daily in close skin-to-skin contact by parent or sibling and given massages, experienced more weight gain and were more active and alert than those babies who were not. It is known that the natural sensory stimulation gained from massage speeds myelination (insulation) of the neurons (nerves) in the brain and nervous system. As the process of coating the nerves (myelination) is not complete at birth, skin stimulation is essential for enhancing the rapid neural-cell firing that improves the brain-body communication and helps the newborn to develop from their primitive reflexes.

Furthermore, loving touch and the oxytocin love hormone boost trigger physiological changes that help infants grow and develop, stimulate nerves in the brain that facilitate food absorption and lower stress hormone levels, resulting in an improved immune system function. As the vast majority of the neural connections in the brain occur within the first three years of a child's life, loving interactions, as in massage, can directly affect a child's emotional development and their ability to handle and adapt to stress as an adult.

Loving skin contact and massage between mums and partners has been shown to help mums during pregnancy; tends to lead to easier and more manageable labours and for mum to be more responsive to her newborns. Touching and handling her baby assists the new mum's milk production, aiding in secretion of the "mumming hormone", prolactin. By regularly massaging her baby, mum gains confidence in her mumming skills day by day and enhances her baby's well-being and their bonding. Research has shown that mums who experienced chronic stress during their pregnancies tended to have babies who cried more and for longer periods compared to mums who were actively supported during theirs. Infants who experience more physical contact with parents demonstrate increased mental development in the first six months of life compared to young children who receive limited physical interaction. This improved cognitive development has been shown to last even after eight years, illustrating the importance of positive interactions. Infants who receive above-average levels of affection from their parents are shown to be less likely to be hostile, anxious or emotionally distressed as adults.

### When should I massage my baby?

Avoid massaging your baby for about 45 minutes after a feed to allow them to digest adequately. Equally, massaging your baby before a feed may not be what they want either. When and how often you massage your baby is up to you. You might give your newborn a massage daily or every other day. Your toddler and older child might enjoy a massage at night as a soothing part of his or her bedtime routine.

Pay close attention to your baby's mood. If your baby has a steady gaze and appears calm and content, he or she might enjoy a massage. If your baby turns his or her head away from you or becomes stiff in your arms, it might not be the best time for a massage.

## How do I massage my baby?

When instructing parents, I am aiming for a basic level of skill that is both intuitive and exploratory as they sense the softening and energetic releasing of their baby's or child's muscles and tension patterns. It's like helping a mum connect with a lost skill that they practised when their baby was in the womb when they would caress and pat their bump!

Infant massage involves a little preparation and here are some basic techniques to get you started:

- **Create a calm atmosphere.**
  Aim to massage in a warm, quiet place — indoors or outdoors. Remove your jewellery. Sit comfortably on the floor or a bed or stand in front of the changing table and position your baby on a blanket or towel in front of you. Place your baby on his back so that you can maintain eye contact. As you undress your baby, tell him or her it's "massage time" - I usually sing the words!

- **Control the depth of your touch.**
  When you first start massaging your baby, use a gentle touch. Avoid over-tickling your baby or child as a rule as it can put them on the defensive, causing them to recoil and withdraw from experiencing the joy of touch. As your baby settles and your confidence improves as you "read" your baby's needs, you can add a bit more pressure to release the tension areas.

- **Slowly stroke and knead each part of your baby's body.**
  I generally direct a parent to start massaging in the buttocks, lower back and legs, areas where the baby tends to be more robust, whilst the baby is lying over a pillow or raised cushion. Then move into the backs and sides of the legs and feet. This will allow your baby to get a sense of your level of touch and active engagement. Mum can also gauge the level of depth and rhythm of her massage strokes and adjust them accordingly as she reads her baby's level of sensitivity and their ability to let go and release tension.

- **Spend a minute or two on each area.**
  Then progress to massaging across the baby's mid and upper back, shoulders and into the arms. Next, place your baby on his or her back and massage across the chest muscles into the arms and hands, thighs and lower legs. Finish off with massaging in light circular stroking movement around their baby's belly button.

- **Stay present and in the moment.**
  Be mindful of giving your child space to listen and sense as to what your hands are doing rather than diverting their attention by over talking. When you feel tension points, pause and hold them and become aware of your breath and gently exhale. Your baby will naturally copy you with practice. You may like to add a word or phrase - "and it lets go" - or sounding a "haaa" may well be enough as you feel the tension release in your hands.

- **Watch how your baby responds.**
  When a child wriggles or squirms, it may be that your touch is either too light or too strong and they need a moment to process it. Re-adjust your level of touch as you stay in contact with the baby's body. Avoid lifting your hand on and off as

you massage as that can be too distracting for a child. Allow all your fingers to make contact with the skin rather than your fingertips and gradually the whole of your hand as your technique improves. Parental touch is reassuring and frequent interaction between parents and baby builds trust and improves baby's development.

- **Know when your baby is finished.**
Babies and children will let you know when they've had enough massaging and will move in such a way that you know they're "done"! However, it's probably best to keep a massage session to a regular 5-10 minute slot so that the baby/child can pace it rather than having a tearful end as the child wants you to continue! Often a parent will notice that they are wanting to complete the massage session before the child.

### Massage lubricant

Either a light, odourless and stain-free massage cream or oil is preferable when massaging. Rub the oil or cream between your hands to warm both it and your hands before applying it to the skin so that it's not cold or, alternatively, store it near a radiator to keep it above room temperature. If in doubt, always seek advice from your general practitioner or community nurse before massaging your baby or child.

Massaging your baby or older child in the evening is not just another thing to have to do before bedtime. As parents settle into this valuable ritual, they also realise how much benefit they gain from this connection with their child at night. Research has shown the value of touch and closeness - something that has been highlighted very much during the pandemic when children have been discouraged from touching and hugging.

I explain to parents that they will have this invaluable skill and tool forever with their children. Parents often comment that their young child will reach for the massage cream and request a massage when they are in need. They may not recognise the emotional reason as to exactly why they need it but they know that they will feel better in their body when they have had a massage. Massaging a child at night before sleep will help them have a greater sense of feeling safe. This is about the child's nervous system regulating itself at the end of the day, a bit like pressing the refresh button on your computer.

Children will often express themselves by downloading their worries from the day during their massage session; when a parent is in a more connected place, they will have more confidence to simply listen and not try to fix and sort out the exact detail of the story that's being told. The child will explain their part of the story, the rights and wrongs, and then I encourage them to wait and listen as the child processes and problem-solves their own steps for resolving it, understanding it or seeking help and advice from their parents. I encourage parents to pace their child - let them unfold in their own way. This is about relational touch and connection that's long-lasting between parent and child.

Sometimes, parents will comment on their lack of massage training and technique and are concerned that they might hurt their baby or child. My encouraging reply is - "But that wouldn't be your intention - would it?" This is an opportunity for you to not only massage your child's tight muscles and to help them stretch out parts of their body where they have been feeling restrictions but also to be present with them, feel and hear them on a level which is very familiar to them. Help your child feel good and you will benefit too.

Some parents will say that their baby or younger child doesn't like being massaged around their shoulders and neck as it seems to hurt them. The parents then tend to avoid touching the area. My explanation becomes an opportunity to help a mum relate to the mechanism of the impact of the pre and perinatal journey that child has experienced; the early imprints that have caused both the physical restrictions and compression in the spine that is still present. This can be a situation where the mum may need help around acknowledging and accepting the child's birth trauma. On some level parents can be in denial and unable to accept that their child struggled both physically and emotionally in the birthing process.

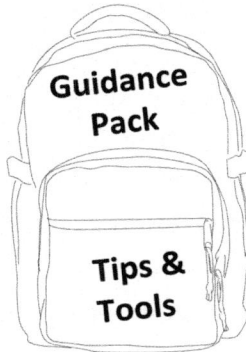

Guidance Pack

Tips & Tools

*"Learn to trust your intuition."*

*Awareness*

**Six takeaways from integrating therapies for children:**

- Learning to proactively manage your baby or child at home is a gift that every parent deserves!

- Engage and celebrate with your baby/child in their first discoveries - for example, staring at you, hands and feet to mouth, rolling over, pushing up on their hands or knees, crawling, sitting up, standing, running, jumping, climbing, swimming, making friends, helping out at home.

- Outdoor and developmental-based play are essential to support your child in meeting their developmental milestones.

- If your baby or child is finding a particular skill set too difficult to achieve then look to an earlier stage of development that needs to be revisited and practised.

- Refer to the guidance on massage techniques to develop your skills and let your child teach you from their feedback!

- Invite family and friends to contribute to your child's "therapy" fund rather than spending money on toys and stuff they may not need.

## Reflections

**As you're now more than two-thirds through reading this book, here are a few things to consider:**

- What is my child telling me that I'm not getting yet?
- Might my child be displaying signs of developmental delay physically or emotionally?
- Am I ready to acknowledge the implications of the impact that birth may have had on my child and seek to address them?
- Am I ready to do some of my own personal development and trauma healing work?

*Remember – trust your intuition as you'll know when the time is right to do this personal work.*

# Chapter Seven

## Challenging Behaviours

In my practice, I observe a trend that as a child gets older and into their teenage years their challenging behaviour tends to become more apparent to relatives, close friends and teachers prompting parents to acknowledge that they need to seek help. The dynamic of the family can be strained by the challenging behaviour as parents and siblings adapt to an unsettled child. Starting from the perspective of 'what happened' to the child rather than 'what is wrong' with them can be more difficult to confront and navigate within this age group. The ongoing unaddressed issues within the family unit may have been allowed to drift with the focus directed towards the child's current challenging behaviour rather than parents understanding and taking ownership of past events. The pre and perinatal issues mentioned in previous chapters need to be considered. The challenging behaviour can be focussed on multiple things from issues with emotional regulation; social engagement; physical and academic ability; preferences around food, sugary drinks, alcohol and drugs; respecting authority and personal boundaries; various types of phobias; separation and social anxieties; attending school, to mention a few.

There is an important link between challenging behaviour and how a child's nutritional needs are met. Essential nutrition is a key factor in the brain development of a growing child as the science around the connection with gut metabolism and brain function is compelling. Children who experience recurrent infections, constipation etc and those who are in need of a boost to their immune system would benefit from a nutritional assessment. It is not within the remit of this book to develop this topic further other than to guide parents to consider their own blind spots in this area so that they can creatively navigate and manage a healthy lifestyle within the family. The next two cases are interesting.

## Daisy - aged nine years

Daisy's maternal grandma, Ruby, had attended one of my Baby Body Language presentations after which she booked a consultation for her nine-year-old granddaughter. Although Daisy's mum, Natalie, didn't think there was anything to be concerned about, she was agreeable for her daughter to have an assessment. Unfortunately, Natalie was unable to attend the first few sessions due to her work commitments. At the consultation, Ruby described her granddaughter as a bright, intelligent child who preferred to sit indoors reading a book for hours rather than going outdoors to play. This was referred to affectionately as one of the family's traits and mentioned as an aside that the Robinsons weren't a sporty family. Daisy was also described as being over-sensitive to criticism and could remain in a sulk for days.

Ruby explained that Natalie's pregnancy had been unplanned and she was not in a personal relationship with the father. In fact, mum had hidden the pregnancy until a couple of weeks before the birth. Natalie understandably had mixed feelings leading up to the delivery but her labour started spontaneously and the baby was delivered vaginally within eight hours without assistance. Daisy was reported as a settled baby that breast fed and slept well but had an accident at the age of two when she fell off the settee and fractured her clavicle.

Since the birth both mum and child had been supported and cared for by Ruby and her husband, the maternal grandparents, which allowed Natalie to return to work as a teacher when Daisy was 18 months old.

Daisy's biological father had part-custody of Daisy, with the relationship between her parents very strained although they did agree on the practical week-to-week childcare arrangements. Daisy was amenable to living between two family homes and avoiding discussing her life in one with the other. She was an astute child who appeared to be very comfortable in the company of adults.

My logical approach in explaining the alignment and symmetry of the spine and pelvis and how it supported the skull and brain immediately captured Daisy's curiosity. As she grasped the relevance of a balanced and symmetrical musculoskeletal system I asked for her consent to assess her postural alignment for optimal balance.

Grasping an older child's curiosity and engagement during the assessment process are essential steps, together with gaining their ongoing permission and consent. A child needs to see the point of attending a session and not just because the parents wanted them assessed. I will pace a child's engagement by stimulating their curiosity around, for example, the simple and logical concept of symmetrical weight-bearing and automatic balancing when standing still.

I guide a child in understanding how their body compensates when I invite them to stand as still as possible and look ahead at the wall in front of them. I sensitively highlight the unconscious movements they are making - such as the wriggling of their shoulders; swaying onto one foot; the slight bend of one knee; or the holding of their breath for several seconds. Usually a child is amused, surprised and curious at these unknown revelations of their body. They are usually keen then to hop onto the bench where I assess them further.

During an assessment my aim is to engage and pace a child's body awareness every step of the way by inquiring how it feels and where they are experiencing any tightness in a muscle or restricted movement of a limb or joint , or indeed a feeling or emotion in their body.

Some children are relieved to share their experience as if they had always known it was there and are relieved to be asked about it as they explain how it feels for them. Others are unable to express it in words but are visibly sensing it in their body as they shift and move, allowing them to process the subtle experience. Parents observing will comment how their child looks so peaceful and relaxed as they too notice the somatic and emotional shift that the child is experiencing.

During the assessment as Daisy lay on her back on the bench, I guided her in anticipating the result of each test that I was performing given that she understood the concepts of balance and symmetry. She found it both interesting and amusing that the flexibility and strength of both her legs were not equal. I explained that her brain and nervous system were protecting and helping her by creating these compensatory patterns in her body. I emphasised that her system was neither faulty nor failing her in any way but that the compensations were necessary to keep her upright. These types of musculoskeletal misalignments and joint restrictions of the spine, pelvic and shoulder girdles and muscle imbalances can be readily corrected. Daisy agreed to engage in working with me to improve her situation.

This approach is essential in motivating a child to practise the recommended neurodevelopmental (ND) exercises and partake in the physical activities which I advise. Children such as Daisy are experiencing ND delay but that's not the language or explanation that I think is necessary to use with the child for their engagement and willingness to catch up although I can explain it in these terms for a parent. Over several treatment sessions Daisy progressed significantly having worked with her from a chiropractic, ND and craniosacral therapy perspective. I guided grandma, Ruby, to direct Natalie on how to practise nightly massages of Daisy's lower back, shoulders and leg muscles. Within months Daisy had progressed from a child who complained how she didn't like walking over "stony ground" and who avoided outdoor play, to a child who fell in love with horse-riding and scooting around on a skateboard whilst still enjoying quiet time in her room to read. In my experience, when you remove the "stops" that are restricting a child developmentally, they will naturally gravitate to the physical activities that are age appropriate and which present a positive and achievable challenge for them. We, as caring adults, need to facilitate that shift by introducing them to these age-appropriate activities.

What is also interesting about this story is that Daisy's mum had thought that she was meeting her milestones in the "normal" way and not in need of any intervention. This was understandable given the family's myth about them not having an interest in sports. Natalie was delighted to see her child's coordination and physical stamina blossom to a level that she had not even considered before.

Many months after Daisy's first consultation, Natalie attended one of my BBL presentations because she was curious and interested to learn more to help her daughter. Afterwards, she mentioned how she had shifted her mindset from the position of wondering when Daisy's early sessions and treatment programme would be completed to a position where she didn't want them to end. She had become open, aware and curious to the possibilities and the untapped potential of the developing child.

Another interesting fact in this case is that Daisy was very keen that her mum share videos of her progress in horse riding, running and playing. On some level, Daisy understood that I heard her silent plea around her "stuck-ness" as I shone the light on her path to self-awareness. Daisy is now 15 years old and has embraced the challenges of secondary school in regard to forging friendships and finding her self-motivation to study and succeed. She lets her mum know when she needs a back and shoulder massage and her six-monthly biomechanical and musculoskeletal with her chiropractor!

## School refusers

Since the start of the COVID-19 pandemic in 2020, the number of children unable to attend school due to Covid-related and other fears increased significantly. However, over the previous decade, I worked with many children who were being home-schooled or tutored due to social and emotional anxieties around attending school. For example, some children found it to challenging to use the school toilets for a bowel movement resulting in them becoming constipated and often feeling nauseated which then led to rising anxiety around any toileting at school and to avoidance around attending school at all.

Many of the young teenagers at secondary school found compulsory morning assemblies, walking along crowded corridors and hurried lunchtimes overwhelming due to the different levels of perceived teasing and bullying they experienced. Some of these teenagers would hide and avoid school assembly without detection, which caused more anxiety and wakefulness at night, leading them to become disinterested in their schoolwork.

Adolescence is a very sensitive time for a growing child as their hormones begin to play havoc, they become more self-conscious, sensitive and emotionally withdrawn with parents often being excluded. One of the first questions I ask the older child at their initial consultation is what they like best about school. "Being with my friends" is the most common reply. Social engagement is very important for young people as it is also a way of measuring how they fit in or how different they are from their peers. Helping a young person to become more physically active and grounded will help them deal better with their emotional and behavioural issues.

### Peter, aged 14 years

### A Mum and Son Dyad

One mum attended with her 14-year-old son, Peter, as a last resort having exhausted every other avenue of support. My first impression, within seconds of meeting and greeting this young lad at reception, was that he was probably one of the most dislikeable children that I had ever met in practice. My next thought was that I should explain to mum right away that whatever his issues were they were not within my professional remit.

By the time we had walked up the short corridor to my treatment room, I reviewed my initial impression and concluded that, as his mum, Patricia was probably dealing with this torrent of verbal abuse 24/7, the least I could do was to listen to her story as I doubted I would make any progress with her son. I invited mum to have a seat on the sofa.

It was difficult to hear Patricia's reply to my introductory questions and small talk as Peter kept up a loud and constant tirade of harsh and disrespectful comments towards his mum: "Why are we here? You're wasting money. You should be working. I don't want to be here. You're lazy. You're fat. I want to buy game X. When can I buy game X?" It was simply a non-stop kind of rant!

I did explain to Patricia that it was highly unlikely that I was going to be able to help her son given his age as I focus on the younger age group but perhaps she would like to explain why she had thought it would be worth having a consultation. Her reply was, "My sister said if you couldn't help me and my son then no-one could..." This comment stopped me in my tracks because Patricia's desperation was palpable - she was at the end of her tether.

Peter continued to prance around the room, like a caged animal trying to escape, as he continued firing questions and comments at his mum. He commanded the room, demanded her attention to reply and every so often would ask, "What's she doing?" - referring to me.

I explained to Patricia that my approach was from a Pre- and Perinatal and early child development perspective. As she shared her emotional story, I suggested that I use some CST techniques on her, to which she readily agreed. I invited her to share her son's pregnancy and birth story. It included a history of a troubled relationship with Peter's dad after their first-born, Peter's older brother by four years, followed by a trial separation and then a failed reconciliation during which Peter was conceived as an unplanned pregnancy. She was a single mum working evening shifts as an auxiliary nurse throughout her second pregnancy, during which her own dad died after a prolonged terminal illness.

Her labour with Peter was induced as Patricia was experiencing high blood pressure in late pregnancy. He was delivered by caesarean section and was bottle fed. Mum reported how Peter was a very unsettled baby with reflux and that she was treated medically for postnatal depression. During this sharing, I supported Patricia by easing the tension in her upper chest so that she could breathe more readily into the lower lungs as I guided her in becoming more aware of her physical body and what she was feeling in the moment.

As her physical posture relaxed and her breathing deepened, Peter asked more specific questions, "What are you doing, mum?", "Why are your eyes closed?" I also noticed how Peter started to prance more slowly and gradually stopped touching and lifting things on the worktops in my room. Patricia then explained that Peter stopped going to school two years previously and refused to have a tutor come to their home. She was currently trying home-schooling to which he had become more and more resistant in participating.

Initially, Peter shouted at his mum for sharing this information with me but she continued and explained that he would spend a Saturday with his dad doing active things like hill walking although he would not stay overnight away from his mum's home. As I guided Patricia in resourcing herself in terms of breathing more efficiently and becoming more aware of her physical body, she was able to describe how she was feeling-weary, tired, depressed and very worried that Peter would not achieve any qualifications by the time he was of school-leaving age. His days were spent on computer games and teaching himself to speak Italian. He also refused to attend the children's mental health clinic after a couple of sessions with the counsellor. Patricia said she had exhausted all avenues in trying to help Peter.

As I continued to focus therapeutically on Patricia, Peter then shifted to becoming more intrigued with his mum. From what Patricia explained, it would appear that life at home revolved around Peter's ongoing needs and demands. Although he seemed unaware of his mum's emotional needs, it became obvious how Peter was dependent on his mum and his attachment issues were being played out in the room. Patricia mentioned how he got very anxious when she went out to work her evening shifts. He would repeatedly check the doors and windows to ensure they were locked and would not go to bed until his mum returned home. In fact, he was unable to sleep alone in his bed and would seek out his mum's bed every night for comfort and reassurance.

I invited Patricia to share how she would like things to be different. She wanted to feel less stressed and find her zest for life. She wanted Peter to work with the tutor as she realised he was academically capable but was unable to apply himself as he got too preoccupied and easily distracted with gaming. I suggested that she hold that intention in her mind and breathe without considering the practicalities of making it possible but to simply "put it out there" and let things evolve. I explained how we cannot change anyone. The only person you can change is yourself. As the session came to an end, Peter snuggled up on the sofa next to his mum, still talking constantly but in a less chaotic way and more in general conversation - "What are we having to eat for dinner this evening?" "Where are we going to walk the dog?"

Mum was emotionally touched and tearful with relief from the unexpected progress in that first session. I tentatively suggested that they both attend again the following week. Peter did not protest or make any negative comments, nor did he agree, but we took that as a positive.

On the next visit, Peter immediately came into the room and sat next to Patricia on the sofa. He had a tablet with him and he wanted to continue playing the game he had bought recently. I went with the flow and asked his permission to place my hands on his upper chest and shoulders in a similar way I had worked with mum on the previous visit. I was able to progress to his cranium without complaint and he agreed to return for another session. By the third and fourth session, we had progressed to Peter lying face down on the chiropractic bench as I worked on the muscles and joints his upper and lower back, shoulders, neck and head. His posture and physical alignment improved significantly, although maintaining any eye contact was difficult for him, and I needed to relate to him via the characters in his video games with the help of my own children's briefings on the subject!

By the sixth visit over a three-month period, Peter was attending the school tutor at the local library and was on course to take some GCSE exams there too. He was less anxious as he was more able to regulate his NS and more interested in life around him. He had found the motivation to apply himself to his academic work. I encouraged mum to become more aware of her language and to reframe the negative comments that she and Peter would use, as she reviewed setting her personal boundaries. As Peter was less anxious, he became more independent and resourceful in calming himself with the odd night in mum's bed becoming the new norm instead of every night. Meanwhile, Patricia had taken more interest in her own health and wellbeing and the family planned to have their first holiday together with her brother and her teenage nephews, Peter's cousins.

The earlier that support can be offered to a mum with a child with challenges, the better, otherwise the spiral effect of disconnection and co-dependency can become apparent with the emphasis then on "fixing" the child as per our health and educational systems which tend to highlight the child's deficiencies, especially to underperformance within the school system.

By learning to interpret and understand a child's BBL, together with offering support to parents, the issues around disconnection and co-dependency can also be addressed in older children. In doing so, parents can then realise that recovery is possible so that they can live with an open heart rather than with clenched fists. It enables them to move on from the grips of fear and discover the depth of a loving relationship that's possible between a parent and child.

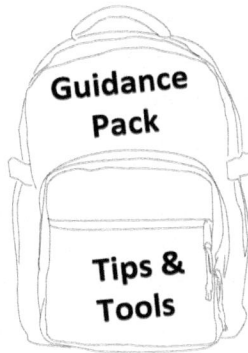

**Guidance Pack**

**Tips & Tools**

**"One day at a time."**

**Awareness**

**Five steps to best respond to perceived challenging behaviour:**

- Notice how you are feeling when your child's behaviour triggers you.

- Breathe! Focus on your breath as you pause, reflect and ground yourself.

- Try to detect the emotion your child is feeling.

- Reframe your everyday language to the positive rather than the negative.

- Remember, our words matter, as does understanding why we may have been using certain body language, words and phrases.

**Five questions you can ask to best support your child:**

- Is your child's nutrition adequate?

- Do they eat regular meals?

- Does your child seek out contact, hugs or deep pressure?

- Does your child chew at their hands, touch or pull at their face, hair or ears?

- If your child is finding a particular skill set too difficult to achieve, what is an earlier stage of development that needs to be revisited and practised?

## Reflections

**Some questions to consider when pacing your child:**

- What developmental stage is my child at?
- Which milestones might my child have missed?
- Where is my child holding tension in their body?
- What are my child's fears or worries?
- What are my fears and concerns for my child?

# Chapter Eight

## Supporting and Guiding Parents

Whatever the hopes, wishes or intentions of any of us as parents, it may be helpful to consider the perspective that a child does not experience the parents; a child experiences the parenting. Let's reflect on this short piece by Dr. Gabor Maté, a psychologist, physician and author who has written widely on child development and trauma.

*"When it comes to relationships between parents and children, it's not just the thought that counts; it's the action that communicates the thought.*

*When we are older and have the capacity to view our parents' behaviour in context, we might find it easier to forgive and understand their actions. However, even that perspective-granted view of events is not enough to erase the layers of belief about ourselves and the world around us that parenting implanted in the first place.*

*This doesn't mean that we need to parent in fear of ruining the children, but to parent mindfully, knowing that we are the single greatest influence that they will experience in their lives."*

*Dr Gabor Maté*

### How could we support parents more?

Parenting can be a learned skill even if some parents think that it's not an intuitive skill for them. Research has shown that planning and preparing for birth can achieve better outcomes for mum and baby. Birth emergencies can and do happen but a positive birth starts with planning and paves the way for positive parenting.

In the therapeutic setting, parents need health practitioners to pause and pace them as they share their child's birth and family stories together with providing support in reframing their language and guiding them through what they are experiencing in their family life. This is what parents should expect and receive. Too many parents struggle through the early days of parenting in need of a guide and in the absence of the proverbial absent baby manual!

**Parents, Julia and Isaac, who we met in Chapter Two, on parental preparation and the benefits of guidance:**

*"They say hindsight is 20/20 vision! It would be lovely to share our experiences in the hope they will help others, we wasted so much time and energy in Tommy's formative years on professionals who saw individual symptoms but appeared to have little peripheral vision.*

*"We now dare to be different and wander off the linear path. We now have a child who can live with us, and we can live with him, not to mention opening a myriad of opportunities for him throughout life. He was so misunderstood by professionals who ought to be informed and trained. They can often have a modus operandi mindset from the viewpoint of their own area of expertise and, unfortunately, coupled with the lack of awareness in the public domain, it can be difficult to navigate a way forward when you meet with issues that you have neither the experience nor resources to understand yet. Guidance is essential when a child is facing the type of challenges Tommy was experiencing."*

The following family's story highlights the notion that our children come into our lives to teach us, as parents, and that in seeking to address our child's issues, we can also become more mindful about doing our own personal reflective work.

Often, we need to pause and consider both the immediate and wider issues that our child's behaviour may be triggering in us. It can be helpful to view the raising of our children as an exploratory journey full of opportunities from which to learn, change or sometimes resist but, inevitably, as we work through the challenges, our various perspectives will shift accordingly.

In my experience, parents often reach a critical point in which there have a realisation that the situation with their child simply cannot continue in the same repetitive and distressing manner. Something has to shift. The crisis point that initiated such a change of mindset can be that last wakeful night of many, or their child having another disturbing meltdown and a parent desperately declaring "this can't continue, we've all had enough."

Interestingly, this critical point is the one that sharply focuses a parent's attention to pause and recognise that the situation with their child has been spinning out of control. This is a call for help from both parent and child to survive family life. This prompts parental awareness, recognition and acceptance that something definitely needs to shift. As this book shows, we need to consider the issue, not only from a different angle but also through a different lens - namely that of our child.

This is how parents Karen and Michael felt when they first visited my clinic with two of their four children, 11-month-old baby Cormac and their eldest child Poppy, then aged six years. Baby Cormac was crying constantly, mum was terribly sleep deprived with just two to three hours' sleep per night and both professional parents were working full-time and at the end of their tethers.

## Cormac aged 11 months & Poppy aged six years

The first step was to help mum and dad in unravelling what may have happened to Cormac as mum related his current symptoms and birth story. After the parents gave the background history, I assessed Cormac and could see that his head and neck movements were stuck and causing him both physical and emotional discomfort. He held his upper body rigid; the joints at the back of his spine were restricted from moving normally which was causing him pain. Mum commented that Cormac had got stuck during the delivery and was born with a tremor-like shaking that had, understandably, led the doctors and midwives to question if she had smoked or taken drugs during the pregnancy which was not the case. His parents revealed that he cried when they persisted with tummy time which concerned them greatly.

Our first couple of sessions involved working gently on releasing the soft tissues and muscles around Cormac's shoulders, back and hips using basic light touch craniosacral techniques together with massage of the buttock and shoulder girdle muscles. Mum reported that after the first session Cormac turned his head from side to side repeatedly on the two-hour car journey home. He was discovering his newfound freedom of movement. Cormac benefitted from the release of the restrictions in his cranium, upper spine and shoulders which had been causing him both discomfort and irritation. These restrictions were also inhibiting him from moving on to his next developmental step. The relief from his symptoms allowed Cormac to get back on to his developmental sequence as he started to practise effortlessly rolling from his back onto his tummy and pushing up on his hands. Cormac's issues were resolved within a couple of visits. In fact, after the first intervention, he progressed to rolling, creeping and crawling and then readily met his major developmental milestone of walking at 12 months.

On witnessing Cormac's immediate progress, his parents were more confident about how therapeutic interventions might help their eldest child, Poppy. She had extremely challenging behaviour, particularly directed at mum Karen, which had become increasingly more and more difficult to manage and leading to family life becoming very strained. The journey to fast forward Poppy's progress would involve Karen addressing her own early childhood story of adversity, grief, loss of a sibling and emotional trauma as she became more aware of the significance of transgenerational trauma.

Addressing our past is a brave and courageous step for anyone and it is the big one that is needed if we want to truly support, nurture and develop the family system.

### Self-care for parents

*"Do the best you can until you know better.*

*Then when you know better, do better."*

***Maya Angelou***

A mum who has had a traumatic birth or has a challenging child, needs validation that they haven't knowingly done anything wrong. In my experience, most of us did what we considered was the best course of action given the information and circumstances at the time. When we strive to become more informed, we will continue to grow and do better for our child. It can be as simple as that; we choose to move forward, with self-love and self-compassion, to a position of empowerment as we advocate for our child. Here are some pointers to help parents and carers re-orientate when feeling emotionally challenged, triggered and not in control of an intense situation with a child.

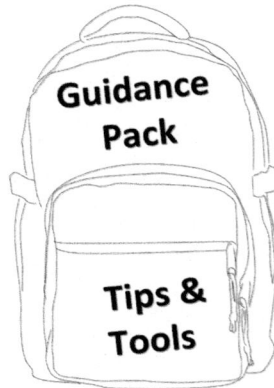

Guidance Pack

Tips & Tools

### The Trigger and Your Response

- Notice what your baby does or your child says that triggers you.

- How do you react to that trigger?

- What is the feeling that is making you uneasy? Fear or guilt? Shame?

- Can you identify the origin of that feeling?

- Notice where the feeling is - for example, is it in your chest or your head?

- Track how the feeling rises in your body as it becomes more intense.

- Practise tracking and slowing down the intensity of the feeling as if you are pressing a pause button on and off.

- Notice, as you slow the feeling, that it gives you time to respond more effectively rather than react as you may have done in the past.

- Continue to consciously breathe out and in as you respond and the feeling settles in your body.

- Notice the mirrored reaction in your baby or child - look caringly into their eyes, pause and breathe out and in.

**Build on your awareness by asking the following questions:**

- Are you doing any body work e.g. daily walking, regular physical activity or home exercises?

- Can you talk about your feelings to a trusted other?

- Do you feel your personal boundaries are being crossed in any area of your life?

- As feelings arise, try to pause and notice your breath - exhale and inhale and then repeat. Notice the feeling dissipating.

- Take care of yourself, walk, talk, laugh but most of all breathe, purposely inhale and exhale.

- Develop your self-awareness.

- Record all your wins for the day, even the small ones, in a gratitude journal.

- Journal your thoughts daily; it doesn't have to be grammatically correct and you may never read them again, nor will anyone else. Just give yourself the time and space to get your thoughts and emotions down on paper as part of a daily practice.

- Make soft, empathetic eye contact regularly with your partner and your child - talk with your eyes more often. Children want to engage with you through their eyes as that is how they communicate and relate with mum and dad; it is part of their social engagement system. Make it regular so that it is not just when situations are intense, when glaring may take over.

I encourage parents to be more attentive as to how they would like their family to develop and grow, rather than focusing on the past and what could have been different. When it comes to attitude and where you want to direct your energy, you have the choice to focus on the positive or dwell on the negative. Focusing on the positive with gratitude will tend to uplift the energy around you and impact positively on those closest to you.

This will help you as a parent to become more aware of addressing your emotional blind spots which are a part of life - but so also is managing them. As you identify these blind spots, practise self-empathy and compassion as you reflect on the emotional journey you've made so far. Allow time to reflect on your progress as a parent and that of your child and, where needed, readjust to where you are heading. There's far less chance of a crash and burn for parents when their feelings are acknowledged and responded to.

**Be open to your emotional blind spots by asking:**

- What am I afraid to hear or know?

- Where did this block come from?

- What am I having difficulty accepting?

- How does it feel being open to change?

### Pause

Take a break from reading for a few minutes and reflect on your thoughts, make notes in the margin or make notes in your journal of what some of your emotional blind spots might be. Please do this without self-criticism or judgement - just with a good healthy dose of curiosity, self-love and compassion!

### Prepare to adjust and move forward

Change doesn't happen all at once. Realistically, you may sink back into your old patterns of behaviour as it is a well-worn path. Don't beat yourself up; be kind and compassionate with yourself as you figure out what it will take to get back on course - then follow that path. I advise all parents to believe in themselves; they can readjust. The above exercises all relate to how we viewed life in the womb and as a baby and the beliefs we were brought up with – yes, it all starts back there!

## Reframing language

Now you are ready to consider reframing your language, your words and your choice of phrases. We have touched on this in most chapters and now we are going to take a deep dive together. Although our words and turns of phrase are creative and expressive, we often take for granted the words we use and do not always recognise that they may be communicating something other than what we really intended. With this in mind, it can be helpful to reflect on how we first learned the words we use and say about pregnancy, birth, parenting and children, and how those words may reflect our family's or society's agenda rather than from a prenatal and perinatal perspective that truly honours mums, babies, parenting and birthing itself.

Taking stock of the words that we use regularly, which can range from sabotaging our own or our child's self-esteem to manifesting what we do want in life, can be very insightful. Being cognisant of our own self-talk is the first step in the right direction of communicating more authentically with our children and others. Consider why so many of us automatically describe our child in a negative way with the sort of phrases listed below. You may have some that you could add to this list:

- She is just a needy child.

- He has a lazy gut.

- It is the witching hour before bedtime.

- She is such a fussy child (especially regarding breastfeeding or eating).

- He is no good at sports, he's a clumsy child.

- My child is a bad sleeper.

- She is so independent that she won't let me help her dress.

In fact, in order to make sense of a situation, we as parents are unconsciously expressing adaptive behaviours to justify some of our own blind spots and unresolved traumas. Commit to exploring your thoughts and feelings with a healthy air of curiosity as if you have a continuous radar system scanning your emotions and feeding them back to you. Building on your work in the previous chapter, journal your thoughts and feelings and sense where in your body you're feeling these thoughts and emotions. Please do not overthink it. The healing process evolves as you notice more of the feelings within your body, overcome the challenges of digging deep and allow the emotions to arise as you're ready to unearth them and give them a voice from your inner child.

### Miriam and her girls

### The Parents' Story

*"I initially went to visit Anne as my daughter was not crawling and I wanted advice in terms of reaching the developmental milestones for her age. I learned, over the next few sessions, many things such as the importance of diet and letting kids explore their surroundings while keeping them safe, as well as that not everything was a quick fix and would involve a partnership between therapist and myself. I taught myself how to massage all my children and the key areas to focus on.*

"My eldest daughter tended to touch her head a lot and seemed annoyed, however, following craniosacral work, I found she slept better and was more relaxed and calmer. Her head was a peculiar shape and, over the coming months, with the help of cranial work, it changed shape for the better and she became less focused on her head and more settled. She also became a lot more mobile very quickly and finally began to crawl.

"I went on to have a set of twins and I visited Anne during my pregnancy. I cannot explain how important these visits were as Anne was able to help align me and work around the two babies in my tummy. I remember leaving my appointments full of the joys of spring yet heavily pregnant. I was much more mobile and relaxed after each appointment. I managed to get to 37 weeks before delivering the girls who weighed 7 lbs 2oz and 6 lbs in weight. Once my twins were born, I immediately booked in with Anne as I knew that both cranial work and massage would greatly benefit my new babies. We discussed areas for me to focus on and I became much more aware of my role as a parent as well as the developmental stages that I needed to focus on. I loved having someone to ask questions to and for those to be answered with options. It helped me to understand there is not necessarily a right or wrong, in parenting there are shades of grey.

"All three daughters have benefitted from my better understanding of their baby body language, and I have chosen to continue with Anne as our guide and therapist. Anne always asks them firstly, if she can work on them and teaches them the importance of their own bodies, how they work and what they need to do to look after themselves. They understand alignment and frequently use ice packs and massage as part of their self-care. Now that they are older and play a lot of sports it is really important that they understand how their bodies work. There is not much that my daughters dislike about the treatments except when getting massaged in areas that are sore or tender and sometimes the giggling that goes on makes me laugh. One of my children is more anxious and I have watched her grow into a much more confident child with the treatments. She has Crohn's disease and is sometimes worried about her tummy in the sessions. We talk about this openly and she is reassured due to the relationship of trust that has been built over the years.

"As a parent, I love the sessions as I also come out relaxed! I again really like the fact that my daughters have someone they look up to and can ask questions as well as understand how their bodies work. The importance of healthy eating and exercise is also something that complements our parenting style! I think the main benefit is that we have happier, healthier children who sleep and eat better and know when they need help or not. Understanding the importance of good food, body alignment, cranial work, exercise and taking care of your mental health are important topics when you are growing up and will leave our girls in a much better place for the future.

"Anne always encourages them to have fun and look after their own wellbeing – something I think we forget to say to children as they grow up in a more challenging world! Overall, I have had a wonderful collaborative partnership with Anne, especially as I had little help from a family perspective and it was so important to have a different opinion and outlook. Anne has taught me to realise that there is more than one way to solve things, to be more open minded and to consider reasons and options that I have within my control. Parenting is not an easy job, and no one tells you that before you take a leap of faith!"

# Recapitulation patterns

*Defined as the apparent repetition in the embryonic development of an animal of the changes that occurred during its evolutionary history.*

We all experience birth recapitulation patterns that were created and computed in our subconscious mind and that have created and contributed to the formation of our blind spots. They were created to help us make sense of our experiences, some of which may have made us feel unsafe, unwanted, unloved, etc. at a time in the past when we were very vulnerable.

Our recapitulation patterns can be either direct or indirect pattern types. In the direct type, we repeat the pattern of behaviour that was wired into our NS and brain as a means of adapting and surviving to our circumstances at the time. "Cells that fire together are wired together" aptly describes the way your brain reorganizes when you have new experiences. The more you do something in a particular way, use words with a specific accent or remember something about your past, the more the neurons that fire together to make this happen will strengthen their connections.

Alternatively, we may have chosen to do exactly the opposite pattern, the indirect type, and are resolute about never having that experience again. Here are some of our common recapitulation patterns:

- You may relive the sequence and nuances of your birth patterns, for example, if it was tough for your mum and for you as a newborn to be birthed. You may have stayed stuck in this pattern and, as a result, developed the belief that you need to work hard to succeed or to complete a significant task.

- You may, in fact, choose to put off doing the task because you perceive the task to be too hard or difficult - this would be a direct avoidance recapitulation pattern.
- You may have the belief that you expect others to have worked hard on the path to success.
- You may be dismissive of those who are successful because your belief is that it is not possible without working very, very hard and suffering.
- If it was hard for you to be born, then you might tend to be of the mindset that you need to work hard to survive, to live and to succeed.

On a personal note, and by way of example, in my case, one of my recapitulation patterns is most obvious when I have to make a dreaded important phone call. This involves doing lots of distracting things in order to put off and avoid making the phone call because I believe and anticipate it to be difficult and yet, when I finally do it, I feel elated and want to celebrate having succeeded. I am often left wondering yet again as to why I was making such a mountain of a molehill around this simple task! The behaviour was wired in my brain and reinforced in my early experiences around avoiding unpleasant feelings, with the result that the behaviour gets triggered and sneaks itself into everyday life surreptitiously. Remember the practice "the pause"; slow down the intensity; become more aware; then re-adjust; adapt to the new sensation as you respond positively.

### Busting more of the myths

The myths I am referring to, are those that are widely held and tend to be false beliefs or ideas. These are the myths that have been built up around our negative emotional states or, to be more precise, they are created from the places where we may be feeling emotionally stuck without quite realising it. We then build our life story narratives and justify our actions and existence from this place of protection. It is an unconscious strategy that makes us feel safe but, although very understandable, tends to be unsustainable in the longer term.

Some of these myths have been cleverly and creatively crafted by us whilst others have been passed down to us from our well-meaning parents, family and friends and so the messy mix of myths continues to be passed down through generations. Now you have an ideal opportunity to clean the slate and interrupt the generational cycle of passing the emotionally charged imprint onto your children.

To summarise, our belief systems have been significantly impacted by our early imprint patterns. Early and first-time experiences that we had in the womb and at birth have impacted our NS. In fact, the narratives and commentaries that we have created about ourselves simply reinforce our original birth story and early imprint patterns within our own stories. We can live up to them; we can make them stick and we can unconsciously choose to repeat them time and time again; our life story script can be very predictable. Alternatively, we can choose not to, and we will discuss that option shortly too.

### Our life themes

Here are some of the bigger themes, or life dilemmas, associated with the various stages of our birthing process and how they are influenced by how we may have experienced our greatest challenge to progress in being birthed. These can relate to the following four key life themes:

- Our state of readiness to move forward in life.
- Our ability to trust our intuition and sense of purpose in life.

- How we anticipate being greeted by others in social situations.

- Our sense of self-worth – am I good enough?

I invite you to allow these concepts to settle with you and you can process as you reflect on the material in this and as we move onto the next chapter. Consider if you have a trusted friend who you might ask to be an "emotional blind spot buddy" and who could help you with spotting some of your life themes.

### Shift gear

One mum described her last baby as "the baby from hell." We had a bit of work to do on reframing that belief, how she had projected it onto her child, how her child was processing that parental belief and how it showed up in the child's behaviour. As mentioned previously, self-awareness and self-discovery can help us make the shift and, as we shed our emotional blind spots, discover our hidden truths and make sense of our old beliefs, we tend to be more open, authentic and emotionally available to our children and personal relationships. We engage and connect with our children on a different wavelength when we resonate with their BBL and, as a result, we have more compassion and understanding to where they are on their emotional journey too.

*"You can't change anyone, you can only change yourself."*

**Anne Matthews**

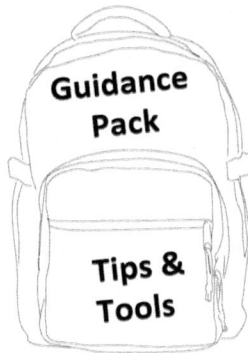

Guidance Pack

Tips & Tools

**"My role model didn't tell me, he showed me."**

**Awareness**

**Six guiding steps for parental guidance. It is time to recap and stack up your parenting backpack!**

- Notice when you're being triggered by your baby or child; pause and breathe, exhale and respond to them rather than reacting without thinking.

- Practise listening more. Listen from your heart as you engage with your child by looking into their eyes as you practise being present for them. Cultivate the art of responding rather than reacting to their behaviour.

- Spend lots of shared time outdoors with your child. Sharing an experience with your child is more preferable and memorable for them.

- Reciprocate your child's sense of awe and wonderment when they share a new experience, learned activity or discovery with you without commenting "I know." Don't be "a know-it-all" parent!

- Remember, parenting is intuitive when we know where to start from and ask, "What is my child telling me that I'm not getting ....yet?" Be a more informed parent as you learn from and integrate your experiences with your child.

- For many families, there is a crisis point that prompts the awareness and recognition that something needs to shift. Do Your own personal work, for yourself and for your family. Be your child's role model of whom they'll be super proud!

## Reflections

**Four guiding principles to live by, consider and reflect on when and /or how you can model these for your child:**

- You do not have to be perfect to be a role model for your child.
- Your child really needs your unconditional love, support and guidance to be themselves.
- Be loving, firm, consistent and positive with them.
- Our words matter, choose them carefully and use them wisely!

# Chapter Nine

## Soulful Connection

*"Our wounds are often the openings into the best and most beautiful part of us."*

**David Richo**

A soulful connection comes from being open to another; to see someone, to hear someone, to connect with someone on a level that is meaningful for them. These are the building blocks for developing trust and rapport in which the other person is being seen, heard and witnessed by you with an air of intrigue, interest and inquiry to understand them on a deeper level because you genuinely care and you want to support them in growing and becoming the version of themselves that they want to be.

We will now consider Baby Body Language (BBL) through the intention of establishing soulful connections within our families, with our partner, baby or child. As you read the pages of this final chapter, I trust that the concepts of interpreting and reading BBL will be fully integrated within you as we share the last few case studies of this book, from an intriguing encounter with a soulful seven-year-old boy, to a mum who allowed herself to evolve graciously as she observed her three sons become more connected and self-confident with their treatment sessions.

### Sean, aged seven years

Sean attended the initial consultation with his dad. A behavioural issue was cited on the intake form, specifically his lack of focus and not being able to sit still at school. When I first meet and greet a family at reception, I direct my attention to the child firstly by asking them if they are, for example, Sean.

I introduce myself as Anne and I then ask them who they have brought with them today. The child usually says which parent or carer it is and a dialogue begins. This is "daddy" "What's daddy's name?" "Seamus" and then I greet daddy.

In the treatment room, I invite the child to sit on the "best side" of the sofa and daddy to sit next to him. By this stage, the child is intrigued with my approach and curious as to what's coming next. I aim to model a manner of engagement that prompts a parent's interest in my efforts to relate and seek a present moment connection with their baby/child by seeing, listening and witnessing their story.

I asked Sean why had he travelled the whole way from Donegal to Belfast. He replied that he didn't know. Most kids will say this, while parents usually want to jump in on the conversation to correct them. As I focus my full attention and animated engagement on the child, parents will generally pause with an air of curiosity as they settle back on the sofa and observe the unfolding of the interactions between their child and me.

I then asked if Sean had visited Belfast before and he recalled that he had been with mum and dad and what they had done in the past, as dad followed my cue by letting him talk. They had stayed in a hotel and had gone to the toy shop. All this is part of the settling stage when a child can orient themselves from the past to now. Some kids' nervous systems are so stressed that they have difficulty recalling past events. This approach allows me to figure out how I can best meet the child's needs as the session develops.

Parents want to comment on the reason for the consultation and usually say something like, "I told you in the car/or last night as to why we were coming here," and often a child really can't relate to that explanation as it probably wasn't that meaningful to them or it may have highlighting their issues which they perceive as bad or negative. Generally, this is something that they are not ready to deal with emotionally at this stage in the consultation.

I often remark light-heartedly to the child that I ask all the boys and girls, "Why are you here?" And do you know what they say? "I don't know." I animate expressed shock and surprise and the child usually titters with laughter as I say, "I just don't know what these parents get up to!"

### Meeting parents where they need to be met

Then I mischievously invite a child to ask their parents, "Why am I here?" This is always an interesting one, as a parent is now in the hot seat; their child is directly asking them the question and they need to choose their words wisely as they have the child's undivided attention at this point. I am curious about the eye contact that is, or is not, made at this stage between child and parent. Some kids will hold their heads down in "shame" or concern that they are going to be criticised, etc, and I am interested as to how a parent deals with this situation as it arises. It also helps me to navigate a path with a parent and to meet their emotional needs, together with accepting their fears and concerns for their child. Some parents attend a consultation with the expectation that their child is going to be "fixed" and they have no idea that they will be sensitively challenged around their own self-awareness and self-development. This is not a criticism of parents; it's just the way that I facilitate change through self-awareness. Usually, parents have been informed by a health or educational professional that there is something wrong with their child - implying that it needs fixing. Other parents have simply been told by another parent or relative to bring their child because I will be able to help without much, if any, explanation as to how I might be able to help them. This is because there has been a trusting connection made between those adults in relating about a child's difficulties and the parent is keen to follow up on the recommendation. I simply build on the connection that initiated attending the first session as a family embarks on the next part of their journey.

With Sean, his dad replied that I was going to show them how to massage him and he revealed that mum is a beauty therapist and was unable to attend the appointment but would be the go-to person for his nightly massages.

I have an underlying curiosity when a mum is unable to attend the first appointment. Any concerns are put on hold as it may well be simply a logistical thing. On the other hand, that is not always the case as often a mum may have been or is still experiencing emotional shock to such an extent that unconsciously she does not want to attend the first visit. She may not be emotionally available to accept that her child has an issue. On the other side of the spectrum, there are mums (with dads) who attend the child's first appointment because simply nothing would get in their way. This is what connection looks like and one that usually wants to be developed further by parents.

## Permission, pacing and leading

At this point, when parents and child have had the opportunity to outline why they think they are in the treatment room, I usually say something like, "Well, what I do is that I help dad understand how clever your body is working ... what do you think?" and I check that both look in agreement and happy for me to continue. I now have permission to proceed having got them both on the same page and curious.

I'm also tracking both the child's and the parents' BBL and how they interact with each other. I'm tracking signs of moments of discomfort or distress, how they regulate themselves, how they breathe, how they listen, how they engage, what defensive strategies they have, their facial movements, their eye contact, how they cross their legs or fold their arms, touch their head, cover their mouth with their hand or bite at their fingers; how they look away, how they engage with me, how easy they find the words to answer my questions, how literally they interpret my explanation, what other paths they go down, if they can allow the situation to lighten up and how I can pace their levels of interaction. All of this is possible as it happens day in, day out, I promise!

I track back on the highlights, summarising what they have told me to date and this allows them to validate their own story or clarify certain points. I loop back and inquire as to how both the parent and child are feeling at various points during a session and repeat what they say before moving on to the next level. This is an invaluable technique in facilitating awareness from an open state of curiosity.

With Sean, I could see immediately that sitting still on the sofa was not easy. He had developed strategies; sitting back into the settee and being very intentional with how he spoke, with how his hands and arms were moving, all aimed at keeping him in one place. Many kids aren't often so aware of their adaptive strategies or so disciplined and will often move their feet and legs randomly; usually parents will ask them to take off their shoes so as not to soil the sofa and others won't. All this helps me build a picture of what and how boundaries are being recognised and managed in family life. I'm not precious about my light-coloured sofa but it certainly helps in giving me some information on parenting and the boundaries around respect of self and others.

Sean was very much toeing the line as I inquired about the activities that he liked doing. Time and time again, he referred to trampolining, proudly telling me how he could do front and side flips and really wanted to be able to do a backflip. Later, I learned that he watches lots of YouTube videos and follows trampoline experts whom he likes to emulate. It became obvious that he was a resourceful child, an astute observer and was very self-aware of his shortcomings which he had sensed were not normal. Surprisingly, Sean was very much in tune with the strategies of his heightened nervous system and with the challenges of his skewed spatial awareness.

I would avail of his resourcefulness later when I invited him to remind his busy parents to massage him at night. Even as a seven year old, I encouraged him to continue with taking ownership of his health and wellbeing by becoming more aware of how he was feeling and by expressing it. I validated the fact that his physical and emotional body were difficult for him to manage to date but that it didn't have to be that challenging nor did he have to feel so vulnerable around his feelings and perceptions of his abilities.

Discovering what a child likes or is passionate about and what they feel good about achieving is key to understanding them. It is easy to list a child's shortcomings; it can often be a challenge for them to list what they are good at. I encourage a child to list all the things that they are good at as I count their achievements on the fingers of one hand and eagerly encourage them to keep listing until I get to my second hand. I will animate this counting gesture with enthusiasm as the child becomes increasingly proud to share with me, from dressing independently to playing ball games, to playing in the park, to helping at home and sleeping through the night. This is the brag list that I encourage parents to focus on.

Sean related how he loved playing tag and running games with his school friends at lunchtime. Learning and relating to a child's social group and including them within the explanation of what I'm planning to do in a session is another worthwhile trust building strategy. Also, I recognised that Sean had a great physical ability and I wanted to tap into it. Some children have very little motivation to run and play; they have difficulty in regulating their nervous system as they have not yet learned the skills, for various reasons, of grounding and discharging the pent-up energy in their system. These are early signs of stress and disconnect well before they become a behavioural or emotional issue.

When I invited Sean's dad to share the "take home" message that he got from the initial visit, he mentioned how emotional he felt after the session for which there were two main reasons. The first was the feeling of guilt around the fact he and his wife could possibly have done something earlier for their child. The second was the unexpected self-awareness his son had and the articulate manner in which he expressed this in the session which had been very enlightening for dad. He also discussed the touching moment towards the end of the first session when his son lay on the treatment bench and I was gently eased the tension from the back of Sean's neck, shoulders and head. We had both observed tears well up in Sean's eyes as he appeared to be going through a moment of inner reflection and emotional release before he reached his outstretched hand and arm towards his dad, positioned in the comfy tub chair at the side of the bench within eye gaze of each other. For a moment, his dad misunderstood the situation as the child being distressed in some way and made a quick-fire reassuring comment, "It's alright …" only to realise that his son was actually reassuring him with a gentle touch of hand holding, full of love and compassion for his dad, which the dad responded to with deep emotion and immediate tears in his eyes. Children can be so intuitive, understanding and soulful and perhaps there's also something around how forgiving they are of their parent's shortcomings and their lack of BBL awareness.

Sean told me that he was looking forward to attending his next session and reported that his parents had dutifully massaged him nightly as instructed, with his mum's skill better than dads! Dad said that he really enjoyed the nightly bonding, that it was good fun for them both and that he looked forward to the bedtime ritual and the quality time with his son. I explained to Sean that I was writing a book for parents on how to help their children and I asked him if he would like to be included in it. After a few minutes of reflection, he said that he would, but only if I told the reader that he really likes Spiderman. So, there you go!

### Parental self-awareness

It has been quoted that one of the greatest discoveries of our generation is that people can change their life by changing their thoughts. We can make a decision to change and reframe the outcomes of how we were born.

---

*"Until you change your thinking, you will always recycle your experiences."*
*Brian Weiner*

---

I am so grateful when parents become more self-aware and are truly present and grounded as they see and hear their child in that special moment. When they embark on this path of enlightened parenting, they are sowing the seeds for deep emotional bonding and connection with their child that is authentic, soulful, unwavering and will last forever. These are also the vital steps towards helping their child develop and nurture emotional resilience as their parents navigate them through their perceived childhood difficulties and challenges, and from which there will be experiential learning and new knowledge will unfold.

The in-between times can be viewed as the mundane part of family life which happens between the pauses that we take to honour our milestones. Without the in-between times, there would be no big moments to celebrate. In fact, it only requires an intention to turn an in-between time into a celebration which we can orchestrate by slowing down, taking time to see, hear and feel from our hearts and take in all of our life's little wonders. Far too often, we can let those simple moments of awe pass us by.

## Our own childhood issues

It is in the raising of our own children, and addressing their developmental challenges, that our own childhood issues will most often come to the fore. A common dilemma is when one parent realises that they are managing the emotional needs of their partner as an adult child alongside their "real child." This underlying co-dependency often first arises when the reason for moving the new baby into a separate room is because that parent's ability to sleep is being overly disturbed. Yes, sleep deprivation is an awful plight when you have a wakeful unsettled baby for a long period of time.

A mum, for example, can get caught up in the emotional dilemma of her partner's needs of preferring to sleep in the marital bed which may override the needs of those of the baby and mum dyad. The situation can be made worse by a partner not recognising nor adequately communicating the fact that he does not want to sleep in another room in good spirit and for valid reasons, but does it reluctantly and in a disgruntled, ongoing passive aggressive way.

The unfolding of this behaviour in a family relationship can be very subtle and manipulative and can be duplicated at various other stages in family life where there is a basic envy if the child's emotional needs are met by an attentive mum whilst a father's envy is triggered. The wife's role then slips into becoming a mumming role with the unaddressed mum/son attachment issues of her husband being projected on to her. Such a mum will often unconsciously prioritise the needs of her young baby until the parental co-dependent relationship reaches a crisis point. As this dysfunctional relationship becomes too overwhelming, and the dad's behaviour becomes toxic to the emotional growth and development of the children, the family unit will also become dysfunctional. Examples of this are evident by how much a father will or will not champion for his child as they grow up. For example, he may be resistant at both parents attending their child's parent teacher meetings; he may not acknowledge his child's achievements; he may not want to support his child's sporting events or hobbies if they don't appeal to him; or, in one example, the father who told his daughter, when she achieved overall first in her year at the end of the first year in secondary school, that she really shouldn't have done that because now there would be an expectation to meet that level of performance in the future. What sort of mixed messages are those for a child or wife?

One wife realised that she was dealing with a husband who had underlying narcissistic and misogynistic tendencies which became more pronounced when the children were in their 20s and were living independently from their father. However, this father had been a product of his childhood, having been sent to an English public boarding school from the age of seven to eighteen and a father who never played football or engaged in rough and tumble with him as a child. It's important that adult children can also understand the impact that unaddressed and unresolved childhood ACEs can have on the mental health of their parents. A parent who uses narcissistic and controlling strategies to disempower others is a parent who probably has their own unresolved childhood issues. It's the responsibility of every parent to be proactive in recognising and attending to their own unresolved issues because, rest assured, having and raising your own children will trigger them and challenge you to do so. A growing family can bring out the very best in parents if those parents take this once in a lifetime opportunity to discover their own untapped potential.

In the example above, it was a brave and courageous act when this mum made a life-changing decision that she had enough of supporting and being drained by the adult child in her life and that her three children deserved more of that parent. She made the decision to separate from her emotionally unavailable husband which, as a consequence, meant supporting and raising her three children under 12 years of age both financially and emotionally alone. She made this decision not knowing how she was going to manage practically in her life but she just knew that the future could only be better than the past. Her children are now three independent, well-balanced young professionals in their 20s whose father has recently estranged himself from them and sadly continues to live with his unaddressed childhood issues.

### Jennifer and her three sons, Aaron, Tyler & Stuart

### The Parent's Story

*"Our craniosacral journey began in 2014 when my oldest son, Aaron, was seven years old. He was due to have several decaying teeth extracted under general anaesthetic and I knew that his diet did not reflect the need for such drastic measures. I moved to a different dentist who suggested Anne to me and she was able to relieve a build-up of acid in my son's jaw. The decaying teeth were never removed, and my new dentist kept them in place until they fell out naturally. My son now has a healthy mouth of adult teeth.*

"When Anne talked to me about the gentle nature of her work and the importance of children being aligned as they grow, it struck a chord with me. I realised that their physical and emotional development would be optimised when their body was able to operate without hindrance. I was so impressed with the work Anne was doing that soon my other two children, Matthew and Samuel were receiving treatment as well. I believe that bringing my boys to regular review appointments helps to negate any damage done by slips and falls and this in turn keeps their posture strong.

"I feel strongly that being proactive in this way prevents minor issues developing into more major ones like the early of release of neck strain, which builds up due to intense periods of schoolwork, carrying heavy school bags or, in the case of one of the children, the strain of carrying a sling for a broken arm.

"As the boys have grown older, and understand more details of the treatment, they are now more empowered to notice issues in their own bodies or to know when treatment would be of benefit. I have also had the advantage of attending Anne and noticed the positives in my own posture and sense of well-being. I am thankful for the way in which this therapy continues to benefit my own children as they grow to be strong, balanced young men."

### Backdrop

When I first met Aaron, Jennifer's eldest son, he appeared to be a very shy seven-year-old who was unable to articulate any feelings of discomfort that he might be experiencing. He had a strained facial appearance with his lips and mouth tightly closed and he had a defensive type of posture with shoulders rounded and pulled forwards. As I worked hands-on, his system was in such high alert that his body began to shiver and shudder under my gentle hand touch as he went into peels of nervous, giggling laughter

248

which he found difficult to suppress. This surprised his mum who gave him a "stop that nonsense" glance. However, as I gently talked and paced Aaron through this physical experience, I guided him on focusing on his exhalations and to notice where he was feeling warm around the back of his chest, neck and head. Mum commented on how she could see her son relax his upper body as I used a simple craniosacral technique of supporting the back of the head as his fascial system in his upper body unwound and he released tension as his NS became more balanced. I continued with the cranial techniques around Aaron's head and shoulders at the next session and he progressed, as mum explained in the testimonial above.

The head, neck and shoulders is a common place for many people where fear and anxiety is held in the body and sometimes these emotions aren't even theirs in the present moment. They are often experiences and emotions that are copied and imprinted in their nervous system. They can be passed down through generations and can be associated with belief systems that are associated with fear, guilt and shame. They simply restrict our children's emotional development if left unaddressed as they hold us back and contribute to the background tension that our nervous system has to deal with.

### Common Fears

*"Feel the fear and do it anyway!"*

*Susan Jeffers*

You may think that you are the only one with a particular fear or that no one else could possibly be afraid of ordinary things such as water, heights, public speaking or flying.

These types of fears are very common and it's well documented about the people who have had great success overcoming them.

Remember, it is not the absence of the fear but the courage to take action despite the fear that determines that personal success. When we learn to face our fears, we learn to observe our thoughts and feelings but not be ruled by them. Instead, we choose how to shape the lives we want and, in doing so, we model that for our children.

---

*"You can't go back and change the beginning, but you can start where you are and change the ending."*
**C.S. Lewis**

---

## Education

### Primary School Principal's Perspective

*"As a headmistress, I first invited Anne into our primary school in 2003 to deliver a workshop to parents and teachers. It made sense to me regarding the physiology and that, if the body is not working properly, a child is impacted on many levels. I had many children at the school who had constant infections or whose schoolwork was being affected by discomfort.*

*"I recommended Anne to one family and was delighted to learn from her mum that one visit had resolved chronic constipation and a recurrent ear infection. A second child had been diagnosed with Autistic Spectrum Disorder (ASD). The child was underperforming within the school, constantly frustrated, and had joined us after a bad experience at their previous school. They were angry at their family, disruptive in class and frequently tried to run away. Anne observed that the child was very keen to do the right*

*thing but couldn't manage it, hence their frustration. They were seven or eight years old and, at their first appointment with Anne, he spontaneously hugged his mum for the first time and in a loving way. The parents came straight into my office on returning to school to tell me of their experience in the treatment room. His parents had been at the end of their tether which, in Northern Ireland, means that they were at the end of their endurance and didn't know where to turn, desperately wanting help for their child.*

*"In school, we observed that their anger had dissipated, he was very calm, and, within a year, his standardised testing scores had gone up dramatically. Here was a child now at ease, both physically and mentally, resulting in him being able to learn, achieve and realise their ability. In P7, just three years later, the educational psychologist commented that he was now overachieving. Many of the children showed a newfound ease or had an issue resolved within a few treatments. Others, like this child, would be verbal when they knew it was time for a visit to Anne for a "top-up!" If I could have got funding within the school, I would have employed her regularly.*

*"I was not able to be in the treatment room with any of the children from my school but I had many experiences of parents calling in to see me after a visit to Anne's treatment room and, of course, my own observations and those of the other teachers of the benefits to the children; from being better able to sit and concentrate to new-found calmness and ease. I knew of the impact, but I didn't know for many years what actually happened within the sessions, that is, until my first grandchild was born."*

## Grandmum's Perspective

*"It was my turn to observe Anne. My first grandchild was born in 2013, we took her to Anne, she had a difficult birth and initially her reaction seemed quite frightening. This little baby was just out of hospital at six weeks old, and she just sobbed and sobbed in the treatment room. Then she eased quite quickly and relaxed into receiving what Anne was doing. There was a big emotional release in that room, from all three of us, mum, baby, and grandmum. Anne also worked with my daughter-in-law, and I remember trying to control my tears. I did hold back in some ways and probably could have released more. It was an empowering visit and Anne gave mummy tips and tools on how to massage and position her baby for ease.*

*"Anne allows a mum to open up and talk about how they are feeling and share any concerns and fears, to know they will be received and responded to in a very supportive way. She has a very calming presence and very high-level observation skills together with great knowledge, intuition, and expertise. Working with the baby, Anne appeared to know intuitively when and where to touch and when to withdraw. My granddaughter had a difficult birth and was very bruised but here we watched her visibly relax under Anne's gentle touch. It is fair to say that, in the few weeks after the birth of her first child, my son and daughter-in-law were a little sceptical that touch therapy could help. After her experience, however, she took her second child and has told me that she refers a lot of friends to Anne, as do I.*

*"I have learned so much and the personal experience with my granddaughter sent me on a personal journey to look at my own birth story and that of each of my own children. I know that I had a difficult birth myself. In fact, I do remember Anne telling me that she observed I had had a difficult birth the first or second time that*

*we met. I didn't really connect with her words all those years ago, back in the early 1990s, but I did understand it the day we took my granddaughter and I cried and cried. Apparently, I cried constantly for six weeks after my birth; I had been a forceps delivery and had to have stitches on both sides of my head. It wasn't until I was in a car accident many years later that I came to learn my neck had also been broken, probably at birth. The car had been shunted and I had a very sore foot and neck the next morning. The hospital x-rayed my neck and there was a tremendous kerfuffle as they said my neck was broken. I just wanted to go home and tell my husband that they must be wrong. The next day, the consultant informed me that it was not a recent break but that I did have a fused vertebrae. I wondered, is that what Anne saw?*

*"So it was visiting her as a grandmum that I came to better understand her magic touch. I have three sons and I know now that all would have benefited from treatment and if I had a better understanding of their BBL. I wanted a natural birth with my first child but, after labouring for 36 hours, she was born by emergency caesarean weighing 11 pounds 8 ounces or 5.2 kilos. I had a very bad haemorrhage, and we both almost died. I later found out that I couldn't give birth naturally and so had to have my next two children by planned C-section.*

*"My eldest son showed so many things in terms of his BBL that I didn't understand. He was always putting his head down and looking between his legs which I now understand was him trying to address the impact of his birth, all that pushing and getting nowhere. He did this until he was about three years old. In the incubator after his birth, all the nurses came to see him as he was so big and constantly putting his hands under and pushing himself up. I now know he was still trying to push himself out into the world!*

*"I feel honoured that my grandbabies are benefitting from this knowledge, and I feel cheated that my boys didn't get to visit Anne's treatment room. I see how the gentle alignment and support ensures that the baby moves forward in the best possible way. Taking a baby to Anne's clinic is, I feel, the very best investment for the future. Better than toys or fancy clothes, these are the greatest gift of all to the parents and baby."*

I would like to leave you here with the knowledge and the tools contained within the pages of this book to create soulful connections within your own family. As this grandmum proves, it is never too late and, whatever challenges arise within our own families, consider that it may also be offering the opportunity to reflect and learn more about the impacts from our own birth story.

To read and interpret both our children's and our own BBL will reveal an understanding of our common reactions and repeated behaviours, especially around emotions that make us feel uncomfortable. Although we do not need to fall victim to our past circumstances, nor should our trauma identify us as a person, there is a wealth of untapped experiential knowledge that sets the scene in the first three years of our life from conception that determines how we live our future. From that knowledge, we can live proactively to ground our nervous system so we can navigate an authentic life path of healing that empowers us to face and learn from our challenges. In doing so, we become positive role models for our children and better placed to assist them in facing their life destiny. It is in overcoming the glitches within our neuro-developmental milestones, both physical and emotional, that we orient more towards the path of our soul's purpose and connect with our authentic story whilst consciously facilitating the same for our children. This is the path to healing transgenerational wounds and trauma.

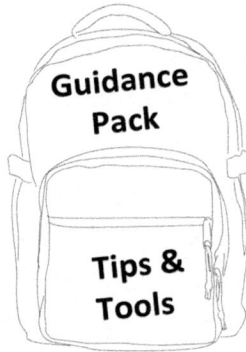

Guidance
Pack

Tips &
Tools

*"It's never too late to heal!"*

**Awareness**

**The Big 12 - Guidance summary for a wholesomely connected family:**

- BBL is an expression of your baby and child's internal state with all their behaviours being a form of communication.

- A child's behaviour correlates with their own parent's neurodevelopment, self-regulation and attachment status.

- Babies and children progress through a sequence of neurodevelopment, the status and pace of which can be interrupted anywhere along the journey from conception in the womb, before, at and just after birth.

- Pre & Perinatal Psychology and Health Education helps us make sense of the impacts of this journey at the level of the baby and child, their parents, their family and greater society.

- The mum and baby dyad needs to be proactively supported and guided from an informed consent point of view, through pregnancy and birth, from both of their perspectives by partners, friends and family members and by professionals who are trauma informed.

- Sharing your child's birth story whilst being facilitated by a therapist from a somato emotional releasing outlook can be a truly healing and transformative experience for both mum and baby.

- Babies and children have the right to be heard, to be seen and to feel safe in expressing their feelings within supportive boundaries created by emotionally available parents and carers, from a wholesomely connected place of empathy, understanding, compassion and love.

- Children and parents all deserve access to a range of integrative health care providers who offer hands-on therapies that help to regulate, enhance and calm the nervous system, improve neurodevelopment, physical ability and emotional balance.

- Among women, traumatic stress from childhood maltreatment often has not been resolved prior to pregnancy and this has implications for intergenerational transmission via biological, psychological and relational pathways.

- Regular physical movement and play, together with shared outdoor activities for both children and parents, promotes connectedness and improves self-motivation, self-confidence, mental health and wellbeing.

- Reframe your language because your words matter. Cultivate responding rather than reacting to your child's behaviours as you practise the 1:2 breathing rhythm to help you become more emotionally grounded and aware.

- Develop the ritual of massaging your child at night before bed, to help release their physical and emotional tension patterns. Enjoy connecting with the child-parent feel-good factor!

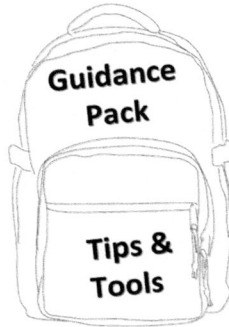

**Guidance Pack**

**Tips & Tools**

**It is time to pass your children their backpack of Guidance Tips and Tools! Baby and children's backpack essentials:**

- Crawling is essential for all babies and is essential before walking. Children still need to practise crawling even when they are up walking.

- For children to dress independently, they need to be aware of all parts of their body and playing body awareness games is essential to be able to dress themselves:

  o Play "Head, shoulders, knees, and toes."

  o Play "Where is your nose, your eyes, your ears, your mouth?"

- Babies will naturally want to be aware of the midline and will clap their hands, touch their toes and touch their mouth. It is essential for crawling, standing upright and walking and to become both more sensory-aware and grounded. The more grounded a child is, the greater is their spatial awareness.

- Physical confidence will help develop emotional confidence. Allow them to use the climbing frames in the park, run, jump and play!

Remember, it is okay if your child complains about being bored - that's when they'll figure out how to do new things.

# Epilogue

## Anne's Story

My mum, Margaret was one of 10 living children of 15, with my grandmum delivering still-born twins in her first pregnancy. She grew up in the 1920s and lived on a small farm with a few livestock and no electricity, running water or toilet facilities. My father, Harry, was raised with his five siblings on a similarly impoverished small farm holding until he was 15 years old, when he was deemed old enough to be sent to work in a prosperous but unwelcoming city of Belfast. It was 1945, during World War 2, and the expectation was that his meagre wages would be sent home to support his family.

My parents had something in common when they met in their early twenties; they were Irish migrants living in another country's jurisdiction which was entrenched with religious, racial and social prejudices against them. The challenge was to navigate these prejudices, both consciously and unconsciously, as they raised their own children against a background of hostility.

I was born six days before Christmas 1956.

If truth be told, it was at an inconvenient time, as the pre-Christmas rush was the busiest time of the year for my parents' thriving off-licence business. My mum also had a "thing" about keeping her pregnancy a secret, although it would have been difficult to hide a full-term bump. This attitude probably grew out of various reasons and myths such as, that good Catholic girls didn't have sex and the often-issued warning – "Don't take your pregnancy for granted."

My mum had delivered her first baby, Theresa, at full term as a stillborn, in 1950, a time when the maternity service within the newly formed NHS was in its infancy. She related how the midwife attending her slapped her back repeatedly with her hand for crying out that she had unrelenting low back pain with her contractions. Harry was then left to carry Theresa's remains alone, in a little white coffin, and bury them in an unmarked plot in the local cemetery as his family did not feel it was necessary to support him emotionally. That wasn't the done thing "back in the day."

I had three older, Santa-believing siblings at home who were being cared for by my uncle, as a two-week stay in the private nursing home, which my mum had opted for after her bad experience in the local hospital, was the recommended recuperation period in the 1950s. However, she had to spend that time alone as I had been transferred to a children's hospital in the south of the city where I had an emergency blood transfusion as reportedly there had been blood in my meconium. Although there was no medical explanation given, I remained in the hospital, separate from my mum, for seven days.

On reflection, my early mother-baby bonding had been interrupted and the negative effect of having a medical procedure without anaesthesia and involving physical restraint had taken its toll. My mother described me as a highly strung and sensitive child who was late to babble and speak. My nervous system would have been triggered and on high alert as a result of the imprints of my early experiences. My mum let slip that a thimble full of sherry helped with my afternoon naps! From the age of six, I had learned to develop avoidance strategies around talking aloud as I was embarrassed and ashamed of the speech impediment I had. The stammering continued well into my adulthood.

I learned to please and help my mum from very early on in my childhood, especially with the family laundry over a twin tub before the days of automatic washing machines. I could sense when my mum was getting worked up and feeling overwhelmed. Like so many children, the caretaker role of a parent starts subtly very early on in life. On reflection, it could be seen that my relationship with my mum was about wanting to make up for that early disconnect, balanced against those early imprints, triggering my survival instinct when I was on my own and all alone as a newborn. I was instinctively aware of my mum's stress and overwhelm levels as I learned that from my life in the womb. Our babies know and understand us more than we realise.

I tended to be emotionally sensitive and, although I could be fearful of speaking and defending myself, I developed progressive and independent traits. My raison d'être seemed to be, life is for living and we only have one shot at it!

The independent trait seemed to trigger my mum who was unaware that our early childhood imprints dictate how we develop and forge our relationships around intimacy, money and food. Transgenerational fear and shame are toxic emotions that can contaminate interpersonal and family relationships.

My mum was a loving and devoted mum who went on to have seven children and often recited the English proverb that children should "be seen and not heard"! Of course, she too was a product of her own birth story and early imprints. Her mum, Mary Anne, who, as shared above, had 10 live births out of 15 pregnancies, had three miscarriages, a set of twins lost in the third trimester and a baby who survived two weeks. Women were just expected to get up and get on with it in the 1900s.

I was raised in a family where there was really no time for open discussion and processing one's opinions on a subject. Instead, matters were seen simply in a judgemental manner of right and wrong with family discussions around sex, intercourse and menstruation simply avoided. As I moved into my teens, I realised a grey area existed which caused friction in my relationship with my mum. Mr Right was waiting for me was as much as the relationship discussion extended to.

Both my mum and father had a strong work ethic and, although emotional nurturing was not a thing, their emotional resilience did indeed keep them together through thick and thin, even within their own dysfunctional relationship until they died in their mid-70s. My father, along with his brother Pat, had been sent to work in Belfast during World War 2, 100 miles from the rural peasant farm where they grew up because he was valued for his productivity as he was known as a hard worker. In fact, the two brothers worked for their board and lodgings for two years without pay in order to pay off a medical debt that their mum had with the uncle they were working for.

Similarly, my mum had been sent into service for a wealthy family in Dublin at the age of 15 and then moved to Belfast when she was 20. When these two migrant workers later met in Belfast, they shared the common goal of wanting to provide for their families back at home in rural Ireland. They married in 1948 and quickly built up their off-licence and pub businesses. Their hard-working ethos was a trait that was valued and rewarded in their own children, often at the expense of emotional nurturing and understanding.

My birth date, 19th December, was a memorable date in the family. It was the date of my father's older brother Pat's birthday. Unfortunately, it was also the date on which he died of stomach cancer at the age of 28 in 1949. Pat, a single man, moved in with the newlywed parents several months prior to his death and, as he gradually became weaker and weaker, they nursed him at home. My mum, in later years, would have described my father as having been emotionally torn apart by his brother's death; his rock was gone and his world was turned upside down. As is the case in so many families, Pat's death caused a rift within my father's family as Pat had bequeathed his only off-licence to my reliable and progressive father rather than to another of his brothers. My parents provided a hub for relatives and friends who were searching for much needed work in Northern Ireland in the 1940s and 50s. They created pseudo positions for them in their own business in order that they could apply for a work permit and then used their connections within the licensed trade to place them in work.

At both their funerals in 1996 and 1997, many of the mourners who we weren't familiar with introduced themselves to me and my siblings. They shared their stories of how our parents had helped them when they were young adults decade ago, such as assisting them to get their first job and, in some cases, to access life-saving medical care in Northern Ireland at a time when the health service in the Republic of Ireland was severely lacking.

Although my parents had moved north for viable work opportunities and then to provide adequately for their own growing family, like so many others, they were not equipped to deal with the civil strife, sectarianism and violence that they were subjected to during the 30 years of 'The Troubles' in Northern Ireland. Violent crime came in the form of petrol bomb attacks on their business which we lived above; the intimidation sale of one of their off-licence outlets; the non-fatal shooting of my brother at the age of 17; the physical assaults on my father; and several bomb attacks of their bar, one of which destroyed the building with my sister being maimed. The death of customers in two other sectarian attacks took their toll and, unfortunately, my father quietly sought refuge in alcohol and my mum in daily prayer.

My siblings and I worked in the shops and bars from our very early teens as was expected in a family-run business. In those days, we lived in constant fear of an attack on the property and worried if a "customer" would pull a gun on us when we turned our back while serving them. On one occasion when the family's bar was bombed, I was leaving through the side door of the building when a pillion passenger on a motorbike threw a detonated bomb into the hallway where I was standing. I had less than a minute to run back in and alert my father and siblings to evacuate the crowded bar were people were celebrating the opening of our new premises. Fortunately, and unfortunately, my sister was the only casualty on that occasion. Later, my father quizzed me as to why I had not picked up the bomb and thrown it back out into the street as that would have saved the devastation that the bomb had caused. I was 17 years old. He was known to have done two such acts of bravery; one when he scooped up a petrol bomb that had been thrown in a similar situation and the other was during the Belfast Blitz in WW2.

In my mid-20s, I moved to Bournemouth in 1982 to start Chiropractic College and to begin a new life distancing myself from the emotional stresses and strains of being an adult child of an alcohol-dependent parent, and away from the fear and anxieties of a fractured and violent society. Although I had a position as a Physiotherapist in a Belfast hospital, on completion of a previous four-year degree, the anonymity and liberation that life at the chiropractic college offered over the next four years set me up both personally and professionally to the extent that I regarded that move as the best single decision I had ever made.

After graduating in 1986, I felt a strong emotional pull to return to Belfast to set up a chiropractic clinic and, at the time, was the only female practising chiropractor in the Northern Ireland. As my expertise and reputation grew, so did my chiropractic clinic. I married in 1989 with my eldest child, Tim, born in 1992, Michael in 1995 and Jacinta in 1996 for whom I was and am immensely grateful and proud. Those seven years were also somewhat of an emotional roller coaster involving the unsolved murder of my ex-husband's close friend in Bournemouth; the death of my uncle to cancer and then both my parents due to ageing related illnesses, together with living with the backdrop of a rise in "tit for tat" fatalities from sectarian shooting incidents and bombings in Northern Ireland prior to the IRA ceasefire in August 1994.

The sectarian issue which I had known all my life became my motivation to do something to try and make a difference in our community. I placed an advert in the local newspaper in 1993 which resulted in bringing together a group of like-minded parents who were interested in setting up an integrated school to educate children, from both sides of the sectarian divide, together. In 1995, Cedar Integrated Primary School in Crossgar opened its doors to 32 children and continues to be a success today.

However, my biggest heartbreak was the delivery of my second son, Philip, as a stillborn at 28 weeks in August 1994. The statistic that about half of all stillbirths occur after 28 weeks and are unexplained became a major motivation of research for me. I embarked on a lifelong journey of self and professional development that brought me into the world of Pre & Perinatal education. I developed expertise in the reading and interpreting Baby Body Language (BBL). I have used my extensive knowledge and skills to help other mums make sense of such loss and to understand the various levels of a baby's distress from the wakeful to the unsettled and colicky baby. Although the death of baby Philip knocked me to the core, a silver lining was that my father told his story for the first time as to how he had carried Theresa's little coffin down to an unmarked grave in November 1950. The small family funeral gathering for Philip gave my parents some peace of mind for the funeral and burial that they had been robbed of four decades before.

In my early 40s, I enrolled on a nine-day intensive residential personal development programme focussed on ridding myself of my parents' limiting beliefs, to allow for transformational change to focus and address my own limiting beliefs. The group participants were required to refer to each other only by the childhood nickname that they had been called within the family. Although my mum's name for me, "blondie bitch", was hard for me to stomach, in the safe environment that the programme provided, I was able to begin a conscious journey of understanding the early stages of disconnect and fractured bonding in the mum-daughter and family relationships. Contradictory messages abounded and yet she was a good woman who was preoccupied with being proud of having good and obedient children. Her grandchildren brought her much joy and I think she realised with age that she had been too strict and inflexible with some of her children.

*"Our parents were guilty but not to blame."*
*John Bradshaw, 'Healing the Shame that Binds You'*

The next part of my journey involved Pre & Perinatal trauma resolution personal work. The focus was to understand and resolve the early imprints that I had acquired in my mum's womb, and the experiences that imprinted on my nervous system from my birth, immediately after birth and in the first three years of my life. This regressive work involved intense somato emotional releasing in workshops and one-to-one personal work over a 10-year period, which is also ongoing. The revelations from this personal work helped me understand my issues around personal boundaries, building and securing trust in relationships and the negative impact of emotional toxicity in intimate relationships.

Just to backtrack, as a 22-year-old physiotherapy student, I was inspired by the French obstetrician, Frederick Leboyer's book 'Birth without Violence'. It just made so much sense to realise and acknowledge that babies are sensitive beings who are very aware of their surroundings - growing and developing in their mum's womb, how she processed her range of emotions, what she ate and how she thought, and the impact of loud noises, bright lights and rough handling at birth. As babies are very attuned to their mums' feelings and energy, the lengthy or abrupt transition during the delivery process of birthing can cause a fragmentation of the connection within this precious dyad, which may not be recognised at the time. This can interfere with the optimal development of bonding and attachment between mum and child.

To deliver and labour a baby in water, which was advocated by another French obstetrician, Michel Odente, was very appealing to me. So, with my pregnancy with Tim, I negotiated with the maternity services of the local hospital to allow me to bring in a birthing pool which I hired in advance, with the attending midwives having travelled to England for a crash aqua-birthing course! Tim and I hit the headlines in November 1992 as I was the first mum to use a birthing pool in a Northern Ireland hospital. I used the birthing pool for my next two labours with Jacinta being fully delivered in water.

Like so many other parents, I had tried, apparently everything, to address the issues around the ongoing wakeful nights that I had with my two younger babies. What I later learned and understood, from my PPN studies, was that Michael, my third child, had been conceived into a grieving womb about eight weeks after Philip had died. My system would have still been awash with stress hormones from grief and I had not received post-stillbirth counselling as that wasn't a thing in those days. I was propelled by a strong desire to become pregnant again as if the propagation of humankind depended on it. Strange really but something that will resonate with many grieving mums in a similar situation.

I also realised that, when I was pregnant with Philip, I had been listening to a news bulletin about a violent crime committed against a young mum who was also at the same stage of pregnancy as me. This poor woman's husband, on returning home, discovered his wife lying dead on the hallway floor with her two young children under four lying beside where their mum had been gunned down in her home. I found this particularly distressing and sobbed at the news which played greatly on my mind. A couple of weeks after that incident, I realised that I had not been feeling my baby moving within and I had leaked water which was the amniotic fluid.

My view of the situation was that my empathetic resonance with this tragedy had been too much for my own baby's developing nervous system, together with the additional stresses and strains that were also going on in my life at that time. Philip did not want to embody this world.

Support of a mum during pregnancy is just as important, if not more, than the mum and baby dyad. It is about setting the scene. The physical, mental and emotional health of a mum-to-be will offer greater outcomes for the developing foetus pre-conception and during pregnancy. The transition of birth will then be seen as a do-able challenge rather than something to fear and to be left in the hands of the medical team to deliver the baby.

This is another myth that many women succumb to.

**"A mum delivers her own baby ... the medical team assists."**

**IN MEMORY OF PHILIP AND THE LOST ONES**

# Acknowledgements

I'm humbled by the children, parents and others who have sought my services and placed their trust in me over the past four decades. They've motivated me to seek more knowledge and develop more skills to serve them better. Also, my deepest gratitude to those amazing parents who shared their heartfelt narratives and those whose valuable experiences I've also weaved into the chapters of this book.

To the dedicated and inspiring teachers and mentors I've had over the years from the various therapeutic disciplines that I practise. They opened my eyes to another world of understanding and connection. This allowed me to be more curious and progressive in developing my intuitive approach to a wholesome and connected way of treating and managing babies, children and pregnant mums.

To my dearest friends and family who have supported me in so many, many ways. I'm especially grateful to those who gave their time and valuable feedback at the critical stages in the process of writing this book, namely - Aisling Cowan, Rachel Jones, Alison Patterson, Aileen O'Kane, Karlton Terry, Claire Murray, Hilary Bright, Claire Gordon, Eamonn Kerr, Heather Shields and Lorraine O'Brien Glenn. Please forgive me for anyone else I have mistakenly overlooked.

Many thanks to the illustrator, Chiho Tang of Oranga Creative and the talented diagram designer, Jacinta Hamley.

My gratitude to my thoughtful and proficient editor, June Russell-Alexander of Russell-Alexander Publishing, who believed in me.

And last but not least, to my three amazing children, Tim, Michael and Jacinta, who have taught me so much around parenting and moulded me into the person I am today. Thanks for sharing this extraordinary journey with me.

# Bibliography

This bibliography is shared in honour of the books, journals and research that have informed my journey, my work, and the writing of this book. If you would like to further your knowledge in any area that has resonated with you within this book, I encourage you to start here.

**In alphabetical order by author:**

**Australian College of Chiropractic Paediatrics**: Chiropractic Evidence Based Management of Breast-Feeding Difficulty Committee on Breast-Feeding Difficulty. 2018

**Alcantara J. & Anderson R. 2008.** Chiropractic care of a pediatric patient with symptoms associated with gastroesophageal reflux disease, fuss-cry irritability with sleep disorder syndrome and irritable infant syndrome of musculoskeletal origin. The Journal of the Canadian Chiropractic Association, 52(4), pp.248–255.

**Angoules A.G. 2013.** Congenital Muscular Torticollis: An Overview. Journal of General Practice, 01(01).

**Anrig C.A. & Plaugher G., 2011.** Pediatric Chiropractic, Lippincott Williams & Wilkins.

**Ashton-Miller J.A. & DeLancey J.O.L. 2009.** On the Biomechanics of Vaginal Birth and Common Sequelae. Annual Review of Biomedical Engineering, 11(1), pp.163–176.

**Bellebaum C. & Daum I. 2007.** Cerebellar involvement in executive control. The Cerebellum, 6(3), pp.184–192.

**Boutsi E.A. & Tatakis D.N. 2011.** Maxillary labial frenum attachment in children. International journal of paediatric dentistry, 21(4), pp.284–288.

**Bradshaw John. 1988.** Healing the Shame That Binds You. Florida. Health Communications

**Brennan B A. 1988.** Hands of Light: A Guide to Healing Through the Human Energy Field. New York. Bantam Books

**Brown A. & Jordan S. 2012.** Impact of birth complications on breastfeeding duration: an internet survey. Journal of advanced nursing, 69(4), pp.828–839.

**Brown C.R.L. et al. 2014.** Factors influencing the reasons why mums stop breastfeeding. Canadian journal of public health, 105(3), pp.179–85.

**Campbell-McBride N. 2010.** Gut and Psychology Syndrome. Cambridge. UK. Medinform Publishing.

**Capute A.J. et al. 1984.** Primitive reflex profile: a quantitation of primitive reflexes in infancy. Developmental Medicine & Child Neurology, 26(3), pp.375–383

**Castellino R. 2021.** Being with Newborns: An Introduction to Somatotropic Therapy® Attention to the Newborn: Healing Betrayal, New Hope for Prevention of Violence. Journal of Prenatal and Perinatal Psychology and Health 35(3), Fall 2021

**Chamberlain D. 2013.** Windows to the Womb: Revealing the Conscious Baby from Conception to Birth. Berkeley, CA: North Atlantic Books

**Colson S.D., Meek J.H. & Hawdon J.M. 2008.** Optimal positions for the release of primitive neonatal reflexes stimulating breastfeeding. Early Human Development, 84(7), pp.441–449.

**Cornall D. 2011.** A review of the breastfeeding literature relevant to osteopathic practice. International Journal of Osteopathic Medicine, 14(2), pp.61–66.

**Cozolino L. 2002.** The Neuroscience of Psychotherapy: Healing the Social Brain. 3rd Edition. New York. W.W. Norton& Company

**Dana D. 2020.** Polyvagal Exercises for Safety and Connection: 50 Client-Centered Practices. First Edition. New York: W. W. Norton and Company

**Davies N.J. & Fallon J.M., 2010.** Chiropractic Pediatrics, Churchill Livingstone. Debes, A.K. et al., 2013.

**Davis-Floyd R. et al. 2009.** Birth Models That Work. Berkeley, CA. University of California

**De Thierry B. 2019.** The Simple Guide to Understanding Shame in Children: What It Is, What Helps and How to Prevent Further Stress or Trauma. London. Jessica Kingsley

**Drobbin D. & Stallman J. 2015.** Resolution of Breastfeeding and Latching Difficulty Following Subluxation Based Chiropractic Care: Case Report and Review of the Literature. J. Pediatric, Maternal Family Health, pp.1–7.

**Felitti VJ, Anda RF, Nordenberg D, Williamson DF, Spitz AM, Edwards V, et al. (May 1998).** "Relationship of childhood abuse and household dysfunction to many of the leading causes of death in adults. The Adverse Childhood Experiences (ACE) Study." *American Journal of Preventive Medicine.* **14** (4): 245–258

**Ferranti M., Alcantara J. & Adkins M. 2016.** Resolution of breastfeeding difficulties and plagiocephaly in an infant undergoing chiropractic care. Journal of Pediatric, Maternal and Family Health. Volume 2016.

**Gibbons T.E. et al. 2011.** Non-IgE-Mediated Cow Milk Allergy Is Linked to Early Childhood Clusters of Commonly Seen Illnesses. Clinical pediatrics, 51(4), pp.337–344.

**Goddard Sally. 2002.** Reflexes, Learning and Behaviour: A Window Into the Child's Mind. A non-invasive approach to solving learning and behavior problems. Eugene, Oregon. Fern Ridge Press

**Grace T. et al. 2017.** Breastfeeding and motor development: A longitudinal cohort study. Human Movement Science, 51, pp.9–16.

**Holleman A.C., Nee J. & Knaap S.F.C. 2011.** Chiropractic management of breast-feeding difficulties: a case report. Journal of Chiropractic Medicine, 10(3), pp.199–203

**Jonas W, Wiklund I, Nissen E, Ransjo-Arvidson A, Uvnas-Moberg K.** Newborn skin temperature two days postpartum during breastfeeding related to different labour ward practices. Early Hum Dev. 2007;83(1):55–62.

**Kain K L., Terrell S. 2018.** Nurturing Resilience: Helping Clients Move Forward from Developmental Trauma. An Integrative Somatic Approach. Berkeley, CA: North Atlantic Books

**Kalef Mia. 2014.** The Secret Life of Babies: How our Prebirth and Birth Experiences Shape our World. Berkeley, CA: North Atlantic Books

**Kalef Mia. 2018.** It's Never Too Late: Healing Prebirth and Birth at any age. Denman Island, BC. Canada. Red Alder

**Karr-Morse R., Wiley M S. 2012.** Sacred Sick: The Role of Childhood Trauma in Adult Disease. New York. Basic Books

**Kendall-Tackett K.A., 2007.** Violence Against Women and the Perinatal Period. Trauma, Violence, & Abuse, 8(3), p.344.

**Klaus M. H., Kennell, J H., Klaus P H. 1995.** Bonding: Building the Foundations of Secure Attachment and Independence. A Merloyd Lawrence Book

**Koch L. 2019.** Stalking Wild Psoas: Embodying Your Core Intelligence. Berkeley, CA: North Atlantic Books

**Leboyer F. 1991.** Birth Without Violence: The book that revolutionised the way we bring up our children. London: Mandarin Paperbacks

**Lelic D. et al. 2016.** Manipulation of Dysfunctional Spinal Joints Affects Sensorimotor Integration in the Prefrontal Cortex: A Brain Source Localization Study. Neural Plasticity, 2016(8), pp.1–9.

**Levine P A. 2015.** Trauma and Memory: Brain and Body in a Search for the Living Past. A Practical Guide for Understanding and Working with Traumatic Memory. Berkeley, CA. North Atlantic Books

**Matthews A. 2021.** The importance of therapeutic presence for the pediatric chiropractor: "getting into right relationship." Journal of Clinical Chiropractic Pediatrics, 20 (1), pp.1740 - 1745.

**Miller J.E. et al. 2009.** Contribution of chiropractic therapy to resolving suboptimal breastfeeding: a case series of 114 infants. Journal of manipulative and physiological therapeutics, 32(8), pp.670–674.

**Miller J.E., Newell D. & Bolton J.E. 2012.** Efficacy of chiropractic manual therapy on infant colic: a pragmatic single-blind, randomized controlled trial. Journal of manipulative and physiological therapeutics, 35(8), pp.600–607.

**McCarthy W. A. 2012.** Welcoming Consciousness. Supporting Babies' Wholeness from the Beginning of Life. An Integrated Model of Early Development. Santa Barbara, CA. Wondrous Beginnings

**McClure, V. 2001.** Infant Massage: A Handbook for Loving Parents. London: Souvenir Press

**Neu J, Rushing J. 2011.** Cesarean versus vaginal delivery: long-term infant outcomes and the hygiene hypothesis. Clin Perinatol. 2011 Jun;38(2):321-31

**Nilsson, Lennart. 2005.** A Child Is Born. 4th Edition. Merloyd Lawrence Book Delacorte Press

**Oliveira, A.C. et al., 2010.** Feeding and non-nutritive sucking habits and prevalence of open bite and crossbite in children/adolescents with Down syndrome. The Angle orthodontist, 80(4), pp.748–753.

**Perry, P. 2020.** The Book You Wish Your Parents Had Read (and Your Children Will be Glad That You Did). New York. Pamela Dornan Books Life

**Porges, S W. 2011.** The Pocket Guide to The Polyvagal Theory: The Transformative Power of Feeling Safe. New York: W. W. Norton and Company

**Rothschild, Babette. 2000.** The Body Remembers: The Psychophysiology of Trauma and Trauma Treatment. New York: W. W. Norton and Company

**Safari, K., Saeed, A.A., Hasan, S.S. et al.** The effect of mum and newborn early skin-to-skin contact on initiation of breastfeeding, newborn temperature and duration of third stage of labor. Int Breastfeed J 13, 32 (2018). https://doi.org/10.1186/s13006-018-0174-9

**Scheans, P., 2016.** Birth Injuries Resulting in Neurologic Insult. Newborn and Infant Nursing Reviews, 16(1), pp.13–16.

**Schultz RL, Feitis R. 1996.** The Endless Web: Fascial Anatomy and Physical Reality. Berkeley, CA. North Atlantic Books

**Scurlock-Durana S. 2010.** Full Body Presence: Learning to Listen to Your Body's Wisdom. Novato. Ca. New World Library

**Seng, J. Taylor, J. 2015.** Trauma Informed Care in the Perinatal Period: Protecting Children and Young People. London. Dunedin Academic Press

**Siegel D J. Hartzell, M. 2016.** Parenting from the Inside Out: how a deeper understanding can help you raise children who thrive. 10th Anniversary Edition. Melbourne. Scribe

**Smith L J. Kroeger M. 2010.** Impact of Birthing Practices on Breastfeeding. 2nd Edition. Sudbury. MA. Jones and Bartlett

**Stewart, A., 2012.** Paediatric chiropractic and infant breastfeeding difficulties: A pilot case series study involving 19 cases. Chiropractic Journal of Australia, 42, pp.98–107.

**Taylor, Kylea. 2017.** The Ethics of Caring. Finding Right Relationship with Clients. For Practising Professionals, Students, Teachers & Mentors. 3rd Edition. Santa Cruz, CA. Hanford Mead

**Terry, K.** Baby Therapy Training Course. Institute of Pre and Perinatal Education. Lecture and workshop notes 2009 - 2012

**Terry, K.** Pre and Perinatal Trauma Resolution Foundation Course. Institute of Pre and Perinatal Education. Lecture and workshop notes 2006 - 2009

**Terry, K.** Embodiment Series. Institute Of Pre and Perinatal Education. Lecture and workshop notes2009 - 2012

**Terry, K.** New Parenting Can Change Your World. More Wisdom - Less Stress. 2022

**Thompson-Hitt, Rebecca. 2012.** Consciously Parenting: What It Really Takes to Raise Emotionally Healthy Families.

**Tow, J. & Vallone, S. 2009.** Development of an Integrative Relationship in the Care of the Breastfeeding Newborn: Lactation Consultant and Chiropractor. Journal of Clinical Chiropractic Pediatrics, 10, pp.626–632.

**Upledger, J E. 2001.** Craniosacral Therapy: Touchstone for Natural Healing. Berkeley, CA: North Atlantic Books

**Upledger, J E. 1999.** Somato Emotional Release and Beyond. Florida. UI Publishing

**Upledger, J E. 1996.** A Brain is Born: Exploring the Birth and Development of the Central Nervous System. Berkeley, CA. North Atlantic Books

**Vallone, S. 2004.** Chiropractic Evaluation and Treatment of Musculoskeletal Dysfunction in Infants Demonstrating Difficulty Breastfeeding. Journal of Clinical Chiropractic Pediatrics, 6(1), pp.349– 368.

**Vallone, S. & Carnegie-Hargreaves, F. 2016.** The infant with dysfunctional feeding patterns – The chiropractic assessment. Journal of Clinical Chiropractic Pediatrics, 15, pp.1230–1235.

**Vallone, S.A. 2012.** Hands in support of breastfeeding: Manual therapy. In C. W. Genna, ed. Supporting Sucking Skills in Breastfeeding Infants. Jones & Bartlett Publishers.

**Van Blankenstein, M. Welbergen UR. 1978.** The Development of the Infant: The First Year of Life in Photographs. UK: William Heinemann Medical Books Ltd

**Van der Kolk, B. 2014.** The Body Keeps the Score: Mind, Brain and Body in the Transformation of Trauma. UK. Penguin Books

**Wall, V. & Glass, R., 2006.** Mandibular Asymmetry and Breastfeeding Problems: Experience From 11 Cases. Journal of Human Lactation, 22(3), pp.328–334

**Wilks, John. 2017.** An Integrative Approach to Treating Babies and Children: A Multidisciplinary Guide. London. Singing Dragon

**World Health Organisation** - Caesarean section rates continue to rise, amid growing inequalities in access

# Return

*"Throw away gadgets. Discard expert opinions.*

*Forget the toys to stimulate intelligence.*

*Don't buy devices to simulate what is real.*

*Return to the real.*

*Connect with your children heart-to-heart.*

*Let them gaze at you, at trees and water and sky.*

*Let them feel their pain.*

*Feel it with them.*

*Touch them with your hands, your eyes, and your heart.*

*Let them bond with the living breathing world.*

*Let them feel their feelings and teach them their names.*

*Return to the uncarved simplicity."*

**Vimala McClure**

**in *The Tao of Mumhood***

Printed in Great Britain
by Amazon

33080814R00159